NURSING DATA REVIEW
1997

Pub. No. 19-7327

Center for Research in Nursing Education and Community Health

National League for Nursing Press • New York

PREFACE

Nursing Data Review 1997 is a compendium of recent research conducted by the National League for Nursing's Center for Research in Nursing Education and Community Health. This volume is designed to be a practical reference book for those interested in nursing's educational statistics. In this publication, you will find comprehensive analysis from NLN's Annual Survey of Nursing Education Programs.

Nursing Data Review 1997 presents data in a variety of forms: the *Executive Summary* reviews the key findings and interprets the data in light of recent public policy trends; *bold graphics* illustrate the data; and *numeric tables* provide the "raw" data for those interested in detailed statistics.

NLN's Center for Research in Nursing Education and Community Health has a long-standing reputation as the nation's premiere resource for comprehensive research on nursing education at all levels of preparation: licensed practical/vocational nursing, diploma, associate degree, baccalaureate (RN and post-RN), master's (generic and post-RN), and doctoral (generic and post-RN).

NLN Research is cited in major newspapers, magazines, and health care publications, from *The New York Times* to *Modern Health Care* to the *American Journal of Nursing*, to name only a few. NLN is also a major supplier of research on nursing education to the federal government.

NLN Research provides information on nursing supply issues, nursing faculty, and nursing students in its other publications, including *Nursing DataSource 1997, Profiles of the Newly Licensed Nurse, State-Approved Schools of Nursing RN* and *LPN/LVN*. Both *State-Approved Schools of Nursing RN* and *LPN/LVN* are also available on computer disks.

For more information on NLN's Center for Research in Nursing Education and Community Health activities or publications, please call 800/669-9656, ext. 160.

Delroy Louden, PhD
Executive Director
NLN, Center for Research
   in Nursing Education and Community Health

TABLE OF CONTENTS

Preface iii

Definitions of Terms xiii

Jurisdictions Included in the NLN Regions xiv

PART ONE • TRENDS IN CONTEMPORARY NURSING EDUCATION

Section 1-1
Executive Summary 3

Section 1-2
Graphs 11

Figure 1	Overall Enrollments Declined for Second Consecutive Year	13
Figure 2	Enrollments Decreased in All Basic RN Programs	13
Figure 3	RN Enrollments to Basic Baccalaureate Programs Increased	14
Figure 4	Majority of RN Students Attended School Part-Time	14
Figure 5	Overall Fall Admissions Declined for the Second Consecutive Year	15
Figure 6	Fall Admissions Declined for All Basic RN Programs	15
Figure 7	Number of Diploma Programs Continued to Decline	16
Figure 8	Drop in the Number of Applications to Basic RN Programs	16
Figure 9	Annual Admissions Increased in Basic Baccalaureate Programs Only	17
Figure 10	Graduations Increased from Basic Baccalaureate Programs Only	17
Figure 11	Modest Increase in Percentage of Minority Students Enrolled in Nursing Programs	18
Figure 12	Steady Increase in the Percentage of Men Graduating from Basic RN Programs	18
Figure 13	Basic RN and BRN Faculty Involved in Various Interdisciplinary Activities . . .	19
Figure 14	Reasons RN Programs Reduced Admissions	19

Section 1-3
Numeric Tables 21

Table 1	Basic RN Programs and Percentage Change from Previous Year, by Type of Program: 1975 to 1995	23
Table 2	Public and Private Basic RN Programs, by Type of Program: 1986 to 1995	23
Table 3	All Basic RN Programs, by NLN Region and State: 1986 to 1995	24
Table 4	Basic Baccalaureate Nursing Programs, by NLN Region and State: 1986 to 1995	25
Table 5	Associate Degree Nursing Programs, by NLN Region and State: 1986 to 1995	26
Table 6	Diploma Nursing Programs, by NLN Region and State: 1986 to 1995	27

Table 7   Baccalaureate Nursing Programs that Enroll Basic
and/or RN Students by NLN Accreditation Status: January, 1996 28

Table 8   Basic RN Programs, by Type of Program
and NLN Accreditation Status: January, 1996 29

Table 9   Mean Annual Tuitions of Full-Time Students
in Public or Private Basic RN Programs: 1995 to 1996 30

Table 10   Fall Admissions to Public and Private Basic RN Programs,
by Type of Program: 1986 to 1995 30

Table 11   Annual Admissions to Basic RN Programs and Percentage
Change From Previous Year, by Type of Program: 1975-76 to 1994-95 31

Table 12   Annual Admissions to Public and Private Basic RN Programs,
by Type of Program: 1985-86 to 1994-95 31

Table 13   Annual Admissions to All Basic RN Programs,
by NLN Region and State: 1985-86 to 1994-95 32

Table 14   Annual Admissions to Basic Baccalaureate Nursing Programs,
by NLN Region and State: 1985-86 to 1994-95 33

Table 15   Annual Admissions to Associate Degree Nursing Programs,
by NLN Region and State: 1985-86 to 1994-95 34

Table 16   Annual Admissions to Diploma Nursing Programs,
by NLN Region and State: 1985-86 to 1994-95 35

Table 17   Enrollments in Basic RN Programs and Percentage Change
from Previous Year, by Type of Program: 1976 to 1995 36

Table 18   Enrollments in Public and Private Basic RN Programs,
by Type of Program: 1986 to 1995 36

Table 19   Total Enrollments in All Basic RN Programs,
by NLN Region and State: 1986 to 1995 37

Table 20   Total Enrollments in Basic Baccalaureate Nursing Programs,
by NLN Region and State: 1986 to 1995 38

Table 21   Total Enrollments in Associate Degree Nursing Programs,
by NLN Region and State: 1986 to 1995 39

Table 22   Total Enrollments in Diploma Nursing Programs,
by NLN Region and State: 1986 to 1995 40

Table 23   Basic and RN Student Enrollments in Baccalaureate
Nursing Programs: 1986 to 1995 41

Table 24   Full-Time and Part-Time Enrollments of Basic and RN Students in
Baccalaureate Nursing Programs: 1991 to 1995 41

Table 25   Total Enrollments in Baccalaureate Nursing Programs,
by NLN Region and State: 1991 to 1995 42

Table 26   Graduations from Basic RN Programs and Percentage Change
from Previous Year, by Type of Program: 1975-76 to 1994-95 43

Table 27   Graduations from Public and Private Basic RN Programs,
by Type of Program: 1985-86 to 1994-95 43

Table 28   Graduations from All Basic RN Programs,
by NLN Region and State: 1985-86 to 1994-95 44

Table 29   Graduations from Basic Baccalaureate Nursing Programs,
by NLN Region and State: 1985-86 to 1994-95 45

Table 30   Graduations from Associate Degree Nursing Programs,
by NLN Region and State: 1985-86 to 1994-95 46

Table 31   Graduations from Diploma Nursing Programs,
by NLN Region and State: 1985-86 to 1994-95 47

Table 32   Basic and RN Student Graduations from
Baccalaureate Nursing Programs: 1985-86 to 1994-95 48

Table 33   Graduations of Registered Nurses from Baccalaureate Nursing Programs,
by Previous Basic Nursing Education and Region: 1990-91 to 1994-95 48

Table 34   Total Graduations from Baccalaureate Nursing Programs,
by NLN Region and State: 1991 to 1995 49

Table 35   Applications per Fall Admission for Basic RN Programs,
by Type of Program and NLN Region: 1995 50

Table 36   Percentage of Applications for Admission Accepted
and Not Accepted and Percentage on Waiting Lists
for all Basic RN Programs, by Type of Program: 1995 50

Section 1-4
Numeric Tables on Male and Minority Students 51

Table 1   Estimated Number of Student Admissions to All Basic RN Programs,
by Race/Ethnicity, NLN Region and State: 1994–1995 53

Table 2   Estimated Number of Students Admissions to Basic Baccalaureate
Nursing Programs, by Race/Ethnicity, NLN Region and State: 1994-1995 ... 54

Table 3   Estimated Number of Student Admissions to Associate Degree Nursing
Programs, by Race/Ethnicity, NLN Region and State: 1994–1995 55

Table 4   Estimated Number of Student Admissions to Diploma Nursing Programs,
by Race/Ethnicity, NLN Region and State: 1994–1995 56

Table 5   Trends in the Estimated Number of Annual Admissions
of Minority Students to Basic RN Programs, 1989–90 to 1994–95 57

Table 6   Estimated Number of Student Enrollments in All Basic RN Programs,
by Race/Ethnicity, NLN Region and State: 1995 58

Table 7   Estimated Number of Student Enrollments in Basic Baccalaureate Nursing
Programs, by Race/Ethnicity, NLN Region and State: 1995 59

Table 8   Estimated Number of Student Enrollments in Associate Degree Nursing
Programs, by Race/Ethnicity, NLN Region and State: 1995 60

Table 9   Estimated Number of Student Enrollments in Diploma Nursing Programs,
by Race/Ethnicity, NLN Region and State: 1995 61

Table 10   Trends in the Estimated Number of Enrollments of Minority Students in Basic RN Programs, 1990 to 1995 62

Table 11   Estimated Number of Student Graduations from All Basic RN Programs, by Race/Ethnicity, NLN Region and State: 1994–1995 63

Table 12   Estimated Number of Student Graduations from Basic Baccalaureate Nursing Programs, by Race/Ethnicity, NLN Region and State: 1994–1995 .. 64

Table 13   Estimated Number of Student Graduations from Associate Degree Nursing Programs, by Race/Ethnicity, NLN Region and State: 1994–1995 .. 65

Table 14   Estimated Number of Student Graduations from Diploma Nursing Programs, by Race/Ethnicity, NLN Region and State: 1994–1995 66

Table 15   Trends in the Estimated Number of Graduations of Minority Students from Basic RN Programs, 1989–90 to 1994–95 67

Table 16   Admissions of Men to All Basic RN Programs, by NLN Region: 1994–1995 .. 68

Table 17   Trends in Admissions of Men to All Basic RN Programs: 1985–1995 68

Table 18   Enrollments of Men in All Basic RN Programs, by NLN Region: 1995 69

Table 19   Trends in Enrollments of Men in All Basic RN Programs: 1985–1995 69

Table 20   Graduations of Men from All Basic RN Programs, by NLN Regions: 1994–1995 70

Table 21   Trends in Graduations of Men from All Basic RN Programs: 1985–1995 70

PART TWO • LEADERS IN THE MAKING: GRADUATE EDUCATION IN NURSING

Section 2-1
Executive Summary 73

Section 2-2
Graphs 79

Figure 1   Number Of Master's Programs Reached 306 81

Figure 2   Master's Enrollments Increased To 35,707 82

Figure 3   Number Of Master's Graduates Continued To Rise 83

Figure 4   Number Of Doctoral Programs On An Upward Trend 84

Figure 5   Doctoral Enrollments Still On The Rise 85

Figure 6   Doctoral Graduations Show An Increase After A Two Year Decline 86

Figure 7   Master's Program Activities In International Education 87

Figure 8   Faculty Involved In Various Interdisciplinary Activities 88

Figure 9   Nurse Practitioner Programs Remained The Most Common Specialty Among Master's Students 89

Figure 10   Nurse Practitioner Specialties Now Offered By 199 Master's Programs 90

Figure 11   Adult Health/Medical-Surgical Continues To Be The Most Popular Specialty In Advanced Clinical Practice 91

Figure 12   Enrollment Of Minority Students Show A Nominal Decline 92

Figure 13   Graduation Of Minority Students Decreased By A Small Percent 93

Figure 14   Largest Percentage Of Male Master's Students Were Found In The West ... 94

Section 2-3
Numeric Tables **95**

Table 1   Master's Programs in Nursing, by NLN Region and State: 1986 to 1995 97

Table 2   Nurse Practitioner Programs in Master's Programs, by Area of
Specialization and NLN Region: 1994-1995 98

Table 3   Enrollments of Nurses in Master's Programs and Percentage
in NLN-Accredited Programs: 1975 to 1995 98

Table 4   Enrollments of Nurses in Master's Programs, Percentage Change
from Previous Year, and Percentage Enrolled Full-Time,
by NLN Region: 1975 to 1995 99

Table 5   Enrollments of Registered Nurses in Master's Programs in Nursing,
by NLN Region and State: 1986 to 1995 100

Table 6   Full-Time Enrollments of Nurses in Master's Programs,
by Functional Area of Study: 1993-1995 101

Table 6A   Full-Time Enrollments in Nurse Practitioner Programs,
by Nursing Content Area: 1993-1995 101

Table 6B   Full-Time Enrollments of Nurses in Advanced Clinical Practice,
by Nursing Content Area: 1993-1995 101

Table 6C   Full-Time Enrollments of Nurses in Teaching,
by Nursing Content Area: 1993-1995 102

Table 7   Part-Time Enrollments of Nurses in Master's Programs,
by Functional Area of Study: 1993-1995 102

Table 7A   Part-Time Enrollments in Nurse Practitioner Programs,
by Nursing Content Area: 1993-1995 102

Table 7B   Part-Time Enrollments of Nurses in Advanced Clinical Practice,
by Nursing Content Area: 1993-1995 103

Table 7C   Part-Time Enrollments of Nurses in Teaching,
by Nursing Content Area: 1993-1995 103

Table 8   Graduations from Master's Programs and Percentage Change
from Previous Year, by NLN Region: 1974-75 to 1994-95 103

Table 9   Graduations of Registered Nurses from Master's Programs
in Nursing, by NLN Region and State: 1985-86 to 1994-95 104

Table 10   Graduations of Nurses from Master's Programs,
by Functional Area of Study: 1993-1995 105

Table 10A   Graduations of Nurses from Nurse Practitioner Programs,
by Nursing Content Area: 1993-1995 105

Table 10B   Graduations of Nurses from Advanced Clinical Practice,
by Nursing Content Area: 1993-1995 105

Table 10C   Graduations of Nurses from Teaching,
by Nursing Content Area: 1993-1995 105

Table 11   Doctoral Programs in Nursing Located in Nursing Education
Departments: 1986 to 1995 106

Table 12   Enrollments and Percentage Change from Previous Year of Nurses
in Doctoral Programs Located in Nursing Education Departments:
1975 to 1995 107

Table 13   Enrollments of Registered Nurses in Doctoral Programs
Located in Nursing Education Departments: 1986 to 1995 108

Table 14   Graduations of Registered Nurses from Doctoral Programs
Located in Nursing Education Departments: 1985-86 to 1994-95 109

Section 2-4
Numeric Tables on Male and Minority Students

Numeric Tables on Male and Minority Students 111

Table 1   Estimated Number of Enrollments in Master's Programs,
by Race/Ethnicity, NLN Region, and State: 1995 113

Table 2   Trends in the Estimated Number of Enrollments
of Minority Students in Master's Programs, 1992-1995 114

Table 3   Estimated Number of Graduations in Master's Programs,
by Race/Ethnicity, NLN Region, and State: 1994-1995 115

Table 4   Trends in the Estimated Number of Graduations
of Minority Students from Master's Programs, 1991-92 to 1994-95 116

Table 5   Number of Enrollments of Male Students in Master's Programs,
by NLN Region: 1995 117

Table 6   Number of Graduations of Male Students from Master's Programs,
by NLN Region: 1994-95 117

PART THREE • FOCUS ON PRACTICAL/ VOCATIONAL NURSING

Section 3-1
Executive Summary

Executive Summary 121

Section 3-2
Graphs

Graphs 127

Figure 1   LPN/LVN Programs Remain Stagnant 129

Figure 2   Adult Programs Increased by 23 129

Figure 3   Number of Public Programs Decreased,
While Private Programs Increased 130

Figure 4   Most Programs, both Public and Private Located in the South 130

Figure 5   Annual Admissions Experienced a Major Decline 131

Figure 6   Decline in LPN/LVN Annual Admissions Also Evident
in Diploma and Associate Degree Programs 131

Figure 7   Fall Admissions Dropped by More Than 5 Percent 132

Figure 8   Decline in Fall Admissions Evident Across all Program Types 132

Figure 9   Enrollments Declined for the Second Consecutive Year 133

Figure 10   Enrollments in Nursing Programs Experienced Downward
                Trend Across all Program Types 133

Figure 11   1995 LPN/LVN Graduations Showed a Decrease Over 1994 134

Figure 12   Graduations Increased Only in Basic Baccalaureate Programs 134

Figure 13   Percentage of Men in LPN/LVN Programs Decline to 12 Percent 135

Figure 14   Increase in Percentage of Black Students Enrolled
                in LPN/LVN Programs 135

Figure 15   Less Than One-Fourth of LPN/LVN Programs
                Participate in Interdisciplinary Programs 136

Figure 16   Why LPN/LVN Programs Reduce Admissions 136

Section 3-3
Numeric Tables 137

Table 1   LPN/LVN Schools and Programs with Percentage Change
                from Previous Year, by Type of Program: 1976 to 1995 139

Table 2   LPN/LVN Programs, by NLN Region and State: 1986 to 1995 140

Table 3   LPN/LVN Programs, by NLN Region and Primary Source
                of Financial Support: 1986 to 1995 141

Table 4A   Administrative Control by Region, 1995 141

Table 4B   LPN/LVN Programs, by NLN Region
                and Type of Administrative Control: 1986 to 1995 142

Table 5   Admissions to LPN/LVN Programs
                and Percentage Change from Previous Year: 1975-76 to 1994-95 143

Table 6   Annual Admissions to LPN/LVN Programs,
                by NLN Region and State: 1985-86 to 1994-95 144

Table 7   Annual Admissions to LPN/LVN Programs, by NLN Region
                and Primary Source of Financial Support: 1985-86 to 1994-95 145

Table 8   Annual Admissions to LPN/LVN Programs, by NLN Region
                and Type of Administrative Control: 1985-86 to 1994-95 146

Table 9   Fall Admissions to LPN/LVN Programs with Percentage Change
                from Previous Year: 1980 to 1995 147

Table 10   Fall Admissions to LPN/LVN Programs,
                by NLN Region and State: 1986 to 1995 148

Table 11   Fall Admissions to LPN/LVN Programs by NLN Region
                and Primary Source of Financial Support: 1986 to 1995 149

Table 12   Fall Admissions to LPN/LVN Programs,
                by NLN Region and Type of Administrative Control: 1986 to 1995 150

Table 13   Enrollments in LPN/LVN Programs with Percentage Change
                from Previous Year: 1976 to 1995 151

Table 14   Enrollments in LPN/LVN Programs,
                by NLN Region and State: 1986 to 1995 152

Table 15   Enrollments in LPN/LVN Programs by NLN Region and
              Primary Source of Financial Support: 1986 to 1995 153

Table 16   Enrollments in LPN/LVN Programs,
              by NLN Region and Administrative Control: 1986 to 1995 154

Table 17   Graduations from LPN/LVN Programs
              with Percentage Change from Previous Year: 1975-76 to 1994-95 154

Table 18   Graduations from LPN/LVN Programs,
              by NLN Region and State: 1985-86 to 1994-95 155

Table 19   Graduations from LPN/LVN Programs, by NLN Region and
              Primary Source of Financial Support: 1985-86 to 1994-95 156

Table 20   Graduations from LPN/LVN Programs, by NLN Region
              and Type of Administrative Control: 1985-86 to 1994-95 157

Table 21   Mean Annual Tuitions of Full-Time Students
              in Public or Private LPN/LVN Programs, by NLN Region: 1994-95 158

Table 22   Applications per Fall Admission for LPN/LVN Programs: 1995 158

Table 23   Percentage of Applications for Admission Accepted
              and Not Accepted and Percentage on Waiting Lists
              for All LPN/LVN Programs: 1995 158

Section 3-4
Numeric Tables on Male and Minority Students **159**

Table 1   Estimated Number of Student Admissions to LPN/LVN Programs,
              by Race/Ethnicity, NLN Region and State: 1994-1995 161

Table 2   Trends in the Estimated Number of Annual Admissions
              of Minority Students to LPN/LVN Programs: 1990-91 to 1994-95 162

Table 3   Estimated Number of Student Enrollments in LPN/LVN Programs,
              by Race/Ethnicity, NLN Region and State: 1995 163

Table 4   Trends in the Estimated Number of Enrollments of Minority Students
              in LPN/LVN Programs: 1990-91 to 1994-95 164

Table 5   Estimated Number of Student Graduations from LPN/LVN Programs,
              by Race/Ethnicity, NLN Region and State: 1994-1995 165

Table 6   Trends in the Estimated Number of Graduations
              of Minority Students from LPN/LVN Programs: 1990-91 to 1994-95 166

Table 7   Admissions of Men to LPN/LVN Programs, by NLN Region: 1994-1995 166

Table 8   Trends in Admissions of Men to LPN/LVN Programs: 1985-1995 167

Table 9   Enrollments of Men in LPN/LVN Programs, by NLN Region: 1995 168

Table 10   Trends in Enrollments of Men in LPN/LVN Programs: 1985-1995 168

Table 11   Graduations of Men from LPN/LVN Programs, by NLN Region: 1994-1995 . 169

Table 12   Trends in Graduations of Men from LPN/LVN Programs: 1985-1995 169

DEFINITIONS OF TERMS

Administrator of Nursing Program—Dean, chair, director, head of department

Baccalaureate Programs

a) *Baccalaureate and higher degree programs:* All baccalaureate and graduate nursing programs.

b) *Baccalaureate and higher degree programs with basic students:* Programs that accept students without prior nursing education. Most of these programs also admit registered nurses who had previously studied at the associate degree or diploma level and are returning to baccalaureate nursing education. Master's and doctoral level programs are also included with these programs.

c) *Baccalaureate and higher degree programs without basic students (for RN students only):* Programs designed exclusively for registered nurses returning for baccalaureate education (BRN programs) and/or graduate education.

Ethnic Background—The categories used to denote ethnic background are:

a) American Indian or Alaskan Native

b) Asian or Pacific Islander

c) Black, Non-Hispanic

d) Hispanic

e) White, Non-Hispanic

JURISDICTIONS INCLUDED IN THE NLN REGIONS

North Atlantic	**Midwestern**	**Southern**	**Western**
Connecticut	Illinois	Alabama	Alaska
Delaware	Indiana	Arkansas	Arizona
District of Columbia	Iowa	Florida	California
Maine	Kansas	Georgia	Colorado
Massachusetts	Michigan	Kentucky	Hawaii
New Hampshire	Minnesota	Louisiana	Idaho
New Jersey	Missouri	Maryland	Montana
New York	Nebraska	Mississippi	Nevada
Pennsylvania	North Dakota	North Carolina	New Mexico
Rhode Island	Ohio	Oklahoma	Oregon
Vermont	South Dakota	South Carolina	Utah
Wisconsin		Tennessee	Washington
		Texas	Wyoming
		Virginia	
		West Virginia	

PART ONE
TRENDS IN CONTEMPORARY NURSING EDUCATION

Section 1-1
Executive Summary

EXECUTIVE SUMMARY

OVERALL ENROLLMENTS IN BASIC RN PROGRAMS
DECLINE FOR SECOND CONSECUTIVE YEAR

According to the results of the 1995 Annual Survey of RN programs, overall student enrollments[1] dropped by 2.7 percent, going from 268,350 in 1994 to 261,219 in 1995 (Figure 1). Associate degree and diploma enrollments declined for the second consecutive year, while basic baccalaureate enrollments declined for the first time since 1988, dropping by 2.8 percent (Figure 2). The decline in baccalaureate enrollments was limited to basic students, i.e., students who did not hold an RN license. Enrollment of RNs into baccalaureate nursing programs increased by 2 percent, and enrollments into baccalaureate programs designed exclusively for RNs (BRN programs) increased by 20.5 percent (Figure 3).

With enrollments of traditional baccalaureate students declining, many basic programs have turned to the growing market of diploma and associate degree RNs who are returning to school. However, when compared to basic students, RNs were more likely to attend school part-time (Figure 4). In fact, approximately 82 percent of BRN programs offered evening classes, and 34 percent offered weekend classes. In contrast, 57.6 percent of basic baccalaureate programs offered evening classes, and 22.8 percent offered weekend classes. Basic baccalaureate programs will need to accommodate the working students' schedules if they intend to increase RN enrollments.

As with the trend in enrollments, 1995 fall admissions[2] declined for the second consecutive year from 96,107 in 1994 to 88,901 in 1995, a drop of 7.5 percent (Figure 5). Fall admissions are used to predict future enrollments. For example, diploma program fall admissions declined between 1991 and 1992, and diploma enrollments subsequently declined between 1992 and 1993. Based on the 1995 results for fall admissions, the decline in enrollments will continue in 1996. In addition, fall admissions to diploma and associate degree programs have been declining for several years. However in 1995, basic baccalaureate fall admissions declined for the first time since 1987 (Figure 6).

Despite declining enrollments, the number of basic baccalaureate and associate degree programs increased by 2.4 percent and 0.9 percent, respectively. The number of diploma

---

[1] Enrollments refer to the number of students who were formally enrolled in a nursing program as of October 15, 1995, including transfer students and readmissions.

[2] Fall admissions refer to the number of first-time nursing students enrolled from *August 1, 1995 through December 31, 1995*.

programs has been declining for the past 20 years, and dropped from 124 to 119 between 1994 and 1995 (Figure 7).

While the number of RN programs increased, there was a precipitous drop in the number of applications[3] to basic RN programs: 8.8 percent for basic baccalaureate programs; 16.3 percent for associate degree programs; and 36.1 percent for diploma programs (Figure 8). This was the second consecutive decline in applications to associate degree and diploma programs, but the first for basic baccalaureate programs.

Overall annual admissions[4] declined by 2.1 percent between 1994 and 1995, reversing a seven-year upward trend (Figure 9). Admissions to associate degree programs declined by 1.7 percent, while admissions to diploma programs declined by 19.6 percent. Surprisingly, basic baccalaureate admissions increased by 1.2 percent, although it is unlikely that this trend will continue based on the findings for enrollments and fall admissions.

In 1995, graduations from basic RN programs reached a new high of 97,052, increasing by 2.3 percent (Figure 10). The increase was dominated by an increase in graduations from basic baccalaureate programs (8.1%), as compared to nominal declines in graduations from diploma (-1.0%) and associate degree programs (-0.1%). Apparently, the trend of declining enrollments in associate degree and diploma programs effected graduations. It is anticipated that graduations from basic baccalaureate programs, while increasing between 1994 and 1995, will shortly feel the impact of declining enrollments as well.

There was a 4 percent increase in the percentage of RNs who graduated from basic programs, and a 25 percent increase in the percentage who graduated from baccalaureate programs designed exclusively for RNs. The percentage of associate degree nurses who graduated from baccalaureate programs increased by 18 percent, as compared to a 1.2 percent decrease in the percentage of diploma nurses who graduated from baccalaureate programs.

For the 1995-96 school year, the average annual tuition at public institutions was $1,984 for state residents and $4,973 for non-residents, an increase of 13 percent from the 1994-95 school year. The average tuition at private institutions was $7,970, a nominal increase of .06 percent from the 1994-95 school year. Private basic baccalaureate institutions had the highest average annual tuition at $10,165, while state residents attending associate degree programs had the lowest average tuition at $1,620.

MINORITY ENROLLMENTS AND GRADUATIONS

Overall, there was a nominal increase in the percentage of minority students admitted into RN programs. In 1993-94, 16.2 percent of the students admitted were minority students, compared to 1994-95 when 17.8 percent were minority students. The increases were most evident in associate degree programs, with a greater percentage of black, Hispanic and Asian students. Both diploma and basic baccalaureate programs had an increase in the percentage of Hispanic and Asian students, a decrease in the percentage of black students, while the percentage of American Indian students remained stable.

The overall percentage of minority students enrolled in RN programs increased from 16.5 percent in 1994 to 17.6 percent in 1995 (Figure 11). In basic baccalaureate and associate degree programs, the increase was apparent across minority groups, with the exception of American

---

[3] This is based on programs that reported number of applications and admitted a class in the fall of the survey year.

[4] Admissions refer to all first-time nursing students enrolled from *August 1, 1994 through July 31, 1995*.

Indian enrollments which remained stable. In diploma programs, there were nominal increases in the percentage of black and Asian students enrolled, while the percentage of Hispanic and American Indian students remained stable.

Between 1994 and 1995, there was little change in the percentage of minority students who graduated, with an overall percentage of 13.3 in 1993-94, compared to 13.7 in 1994-95. In basic baccalaureate programs, the percentage of black students who graduated increased from 6.6 percent to 7.3 percent from 1994 to 1995. Otherwise, the percentage of minority students who graduated remained stable: 3 percent were Hispanic students; 4 percent were Asian students; and 0.5 percent were American Indian students. Associate degree programs had a similar ratio of minority students, although the percentage of Asian students was somewhat lower at 2.6 percent. As in the past, diploma students had the lowest percentage of minority graduates, with 5.5 percent black, 2.7 percent Hispanic, 2.3 percent Asian, and 0.3 percent American Indian.

ENROLLMENT OF MEN IN RN PROGRAMS

In 1995, the percentage of men who were admitted to basic baccalaureate, associate degree and diploma programs reached 13 percent, and represented little change from 1994. The percentage of men enrolled in basic baccalaureate and diploma programs was slightly lower at 12 percent, while associate degree programs was slightly higher at 14 percent. Male graduates increased from 11.4 percent in 1994 to 12.4 percent in 1995 (Figure 12). Across program type, male graduates increased by one percent, reaching approximately 12 percent for basic baccalaureate and associate degree programs, and 13 percent for diploma programs.

CURRENT ISSUES IN NURSING EDUCATION

Each year, questions are included on the NLN Annual Survey to address current issues in nursing education. The 1995 Annual Survey included a wide range of questions concerning involvement in international and interdisciplinary activities, health care settings for students' clinical experiences, students' knowledge of computer applications, and whether nursing programs were planning to reduce admissions.

The overall results indicated that the majority of RN and BRN programs were not involved in international activities. The highest response rate was for "study abroad programs for students" (12.1%), followed by "collaborative research/teaching/training with international agencies or universities" (8.1%). The results according to program type indicated that basic baccalaureate and BRN programs had the most involvement in international activities.

RN and BRN faculty were more likely to participate in interdisciplinary, rather than international activities (Figure 13). Over one-third of the faculty taught interdisciplinary courses, approximately one-fourth prepared research grants with faculty from other disciplines and one-fourth participated in regional accreditation of colleges. In general, faculty from basic baccalaureate and BRN programs, as compared to associate degree and diploma programs, were more likely to be involved in these activities. For example, approximately 52 percent of baccalaureate faculty taught interdisciplinary courses, compared to 23 percent of associate degree and 14 percent of diploma faculty.

With regard to students' clinical experiences, approximately 52 percent of the programs reported that the majority of the experiences were in acute care settings. In addition, more than half of the programs reported no more than 20 percent of clinical experiences were spent in community-based care or long-term care settings. However, basic baccalaureate programs were more likely to provide community-based care experiences, while associate degree programs were more likely to provide long-term care experiences.

With regard to use of computers, approximately 63 percent of the programs reported that their students were most conversant with personal computers, and an equal percentage were familiar with "Windows" as compared to "MS-DOS" applications. These results were quite consistent across program type.

When asked whether the nursing program was planning to reduce the number of students admitted, approximately 25 percent responded yes. The percentage that planned reductions, according to program type, was: 59 percent of diploma programs; 26 percent of associate degree; 21 percent of basic baccalaureate; and 10 percent of BRN programs. Approximately 12 percent of nursing programs reduced admissions due to "lack of perceived job opportunities" and 8 percent due to "budget reductions". Associate degree and diploma programs were more likely to cite the former, while basic baccalaureate programs were more likely to cite the latter (Figure 14). For approximately half of the respondents, the planned reductions were no greater than 10 percent, although a few programs planned to reduce admission by as much as 80 percent.

TRENDS IN NURSING EDUCATION

When viewing nursing education over the past 25 years in terms of admissions, enrollments and graduations, the numbers fluctuated between upward and downward trends. For example, enrollments increased from 1971 through 1975; decreased from 1976 through 1980; increased from 1981 through 1983; decreased from 1984 through 1987; and increased from 1988 through 1993. The recent decline in enrollments could be viewed as part of the normal cycle, and perhaps considered long overdue after six straight years of increasing enrollments. However, this should not stop nurse educators from considering reasons for the decline, and what if anything should be done about it.

In 1995, the Pew Health Professions Commission[1] recommended that the size and number of nursing education programs be reduced between 10 and 20 percent, due to the loss of perhaps 60 percent of hospital beds, which would result in a surplus of 200,000 to 300,000 nurses. As stated in the report,

> In five brief years the organizational, financial and legal framework of much of health care in the U.S. have been transformed to emerging systems of integrated care that combine primary, specialty and hospital services. These systems attempt to manage the care delivered to enrolled populations in such a manner as to achieve some combination of cost reduction, enhanced patient and consumer satisfaction, and improvement of health care outcomes. (p.i)

The results from the 1995 Annual Survey indicate that declining admissions is in fact a policy decision on the part of one-fourth of the RN programs, with lack of perceived job opportunities a contributing factor, especially for hospital-based diploma programs. This is a realistic perception as hospital administrators close patient units, and sometimes entire hospitals, in reaction to reduced patient admissions and shorter length of stays.[2] As recently reported in *The New York Times*[3], five years ago nursing jobs were plentiful in New York, with starting salaries at $50,000. However, now as a result of budget reductions, "...hospitals that once fought one another to attract nurses now see their large nursing staff as costly burdens" (p. B1).

In some cases, RNs are replaced by unlicensed assistive personnel. Many state nursing organizations are fighting such efforts at "reengineering" by focusing on patient safety.[4] Wilkinson[5] stated,

As hospitals struggle to cut costs, they are restructuring patient care roles and using fewer registered nurses. When there are no workers to fit their job requirements, they too are training them in-house—with or without supervision from state boards of nursing or nursing accrediting bodies such as the NLN. (p.72)

However, reengineering has also resulted in a call for nurse educators to re-examine the nursing curricula to better fit the changing health care environment. On the one hand, Holzemer[6] suggested that the nursing curricula should include patient care management in community-based and managed care settings. He emphasized that students need "...to learn how decentralized, consumer-managed health care services are provided" (p.6). Wilkinson[5] on the other hand, suggested a differentiated curricula with four levels of nursing education. Lindeman[7] proposed that, within the redesigned health care settings, the most important outcomes from undergraduate nursing education are now: 1) relationship-centered care skills; 2) care management skills; 3) primary care skills; and 4) community focus skills.

These proposals represent attempts to adapt nursing education to the changing health care systems. Such proposals may be criticized as shifting "nursing education" to "job training". However, other disciplines have also adapted to changing work environments. For example, computer science progressed from mainframes to stand alone personal computers to networks to the Internet. Medicine as well must deal with the change in the health care system which now values general practitioners rather than specialists. If nurses are to continue their work as effective health care providers, they must be able to function within a changing health care system which has altered the traditional hospital-based role, and has included managed and community-based care. As stated by Dr. Lindeman,[8]

There is an old adage that advises, "If your horse dies, we suggest you dismount." In many schools, the nursing curriculum has died. It is time that faculty dismount and create a new curriculum. (p. 227)

Donna Post, PhD
Director of Research
NLN Center for Research in Nursing
Education and Community Health

Delroy Louden, PhD
Executive Director
NLN Center for Research in Nursing
Education and Community Health

REFERENCES

1. Pew Health Professions Commission. (1995). *Critical challenges: Revitalizing the health professions for the twenty-first century* (Third Report). San Francisco: University of California, Center for the Health Professions.

2. Lumsdon, K. (1995, December 5). Faded glory: Will nursing ever be the same? *Hospitals & Health Networks*, 31-35.

3. Rosenthal, E. (1996, August 19). Once in big demand, nurses are targets for hospital cuts. *The New York Times*, pp. B1, B4.

4. Whittaker, S. (1996). SNAs face threats to practice, push quality initiatives. *The American Nurse, 28*(3), 18.

5. Wilkinson, J.M. (1996). The "C" word: A curriculum for the future. *N & HC Perspectives on Community, 17*(2), 72-81.

6. Holzemer, S.P. (1996). Escorting nursing faculty and students into community-based and managed care environments. *NLN Research & Policy PRISM, 4*(2), 6.

7. Lindeman, C.A. (1996). Curriculum changes needed in nursing education. *The American Nurse, 28*(6), 6.

8. Lindeman, C.A. (1996). Professional cannibalism. *N & HC Perspectives on Community, 17*(5), 227.

**Section 1-2
Graphs**

Figure 1
OVERALL ENROLLMENTS DECLINED
FOR SECOND CONSECUTIVE YEAR

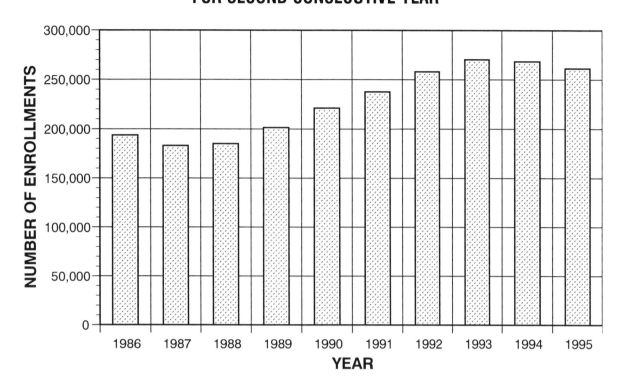

Figure 2
ENROLLMENTS DECREASED IN ALL BASIC RN PROGRAMS

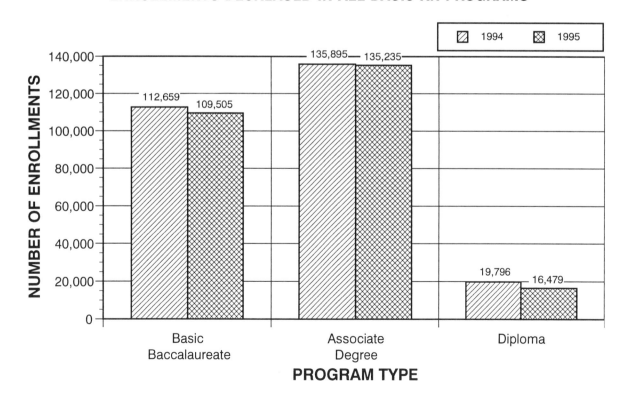

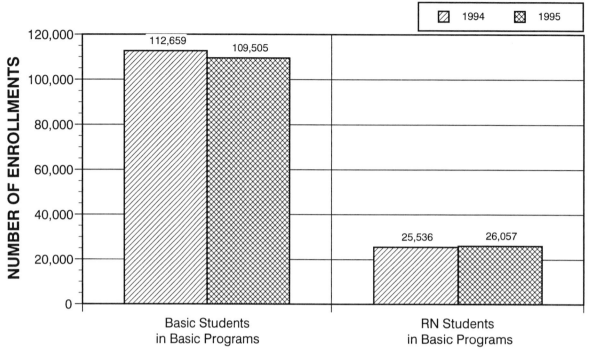

Figure 3
RN ENROLLMENTS TO BASIC BACCALAUREATE PROGRAMS INCREASED

TYPE OF BASIC BACCALUREATE STUDENT

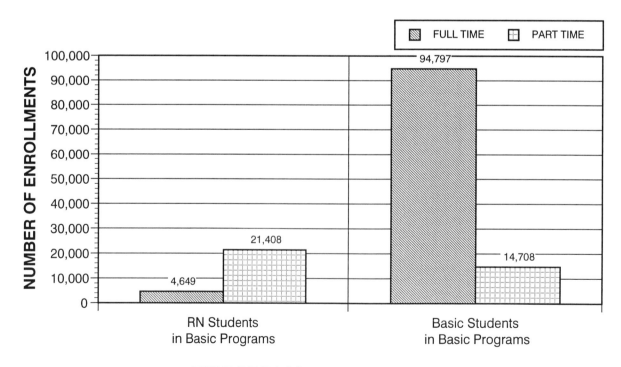

Figure 4
MAJORITY OF RN STUDENTS ATTENDED SCHOOL PART-TIME

TYPE OF BACCALAUREATE STUDENTS

Figure 5
OVERALL FALL ADMISSIONS
DECLINED FOR THE SECOND CONSECUTIVE YEAR

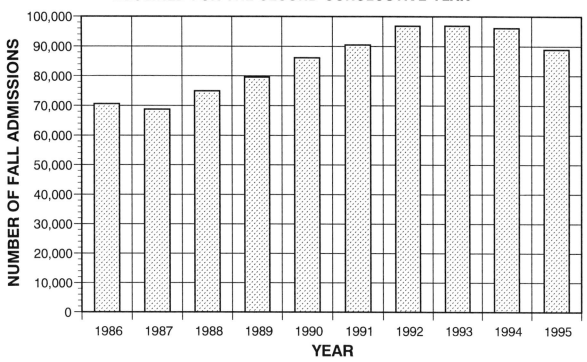

Figure 6
FALL ADMISSIONS DECLINED FOR ALL BASIC RN PROGRAMS

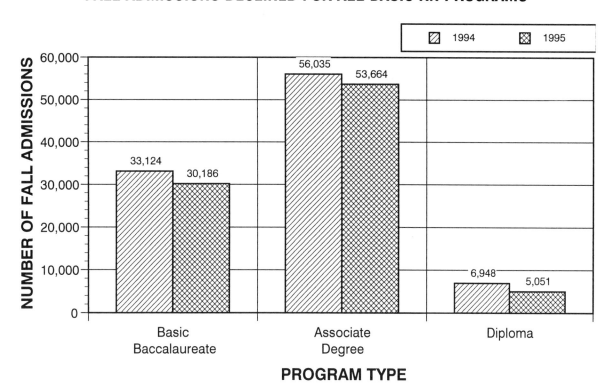

Figure 7
NUMBER OF DIPLOMA PROGRAMS CONTINUED TO DECLINE

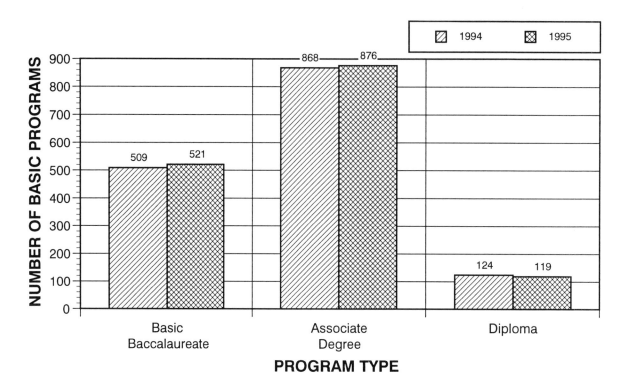

Figure 8
DROP IN THE NUMBER OF APPLICATIONS TO BASIC RN PROGRAMS*

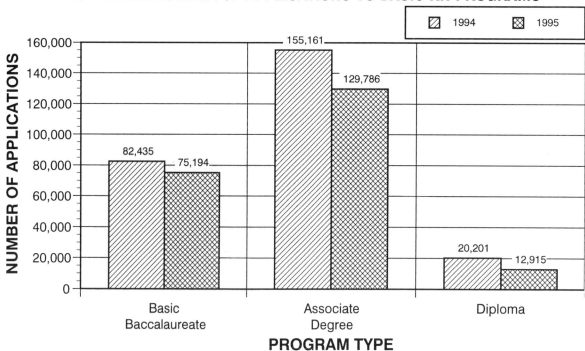

*Included programs that reported number of applications, and admitted a class in the fall of the survey year.

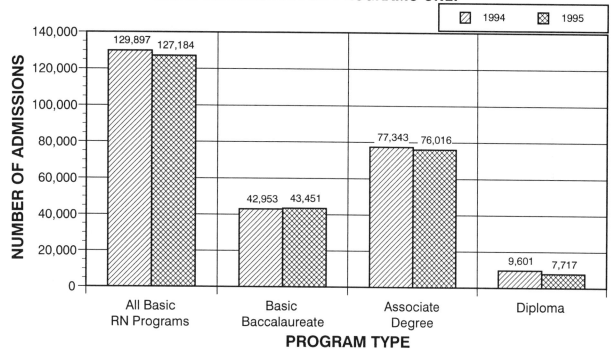

Figure 9
**ANNUAL ADMISSIONS INCREASED IN
BASIC BACCALAUREATE PROGRAMS ONLY**

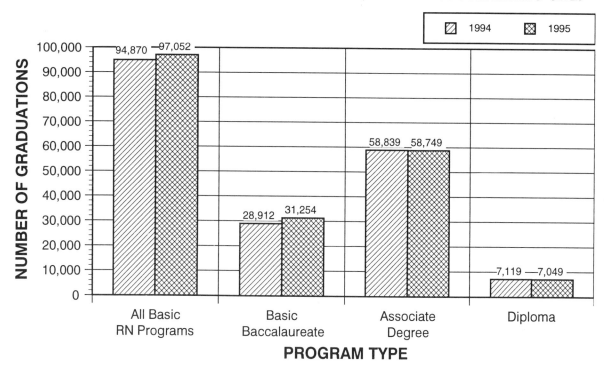

Figure 10
GRADUATIONS INCREASED FROM BASIC BACCALAUREATE PROGRAMS ONLY

17

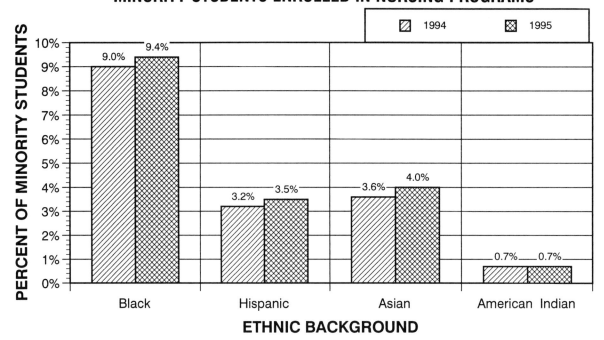

Figure 11
MODEST INCREASE IN PERCENTAGE OF
MINORITY STUDENTS ENROLLED IN NURSING PROGRAMS

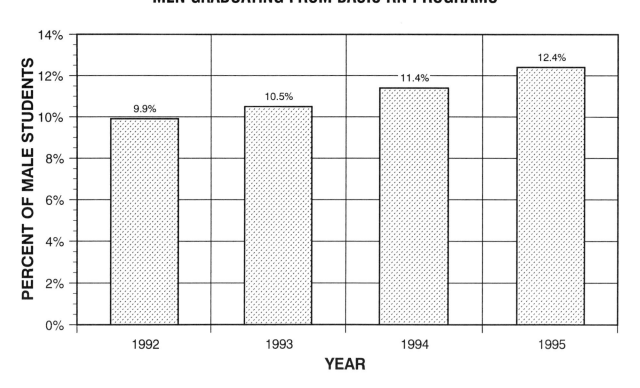

Figure 12
STEADY INCREASE IN THE PERCENTAGE OF
MEN GRADUATING FROM BASIC RN PROGRAMS

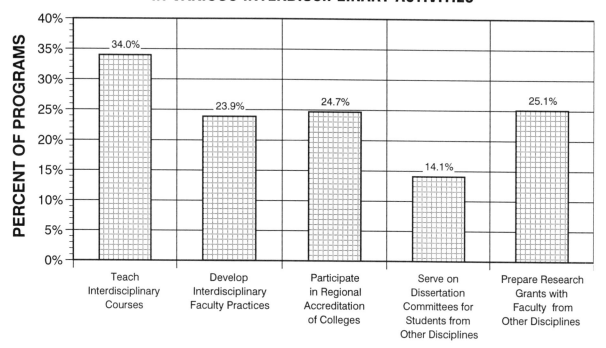

Figure 13
BASIC RN AND BRN FACULTY INVOLVED
IN VARIOUS INTERDISCIPLINARY ACTIVITIES

TYPE OF INTERDISCIPLINARY ACTIVITY

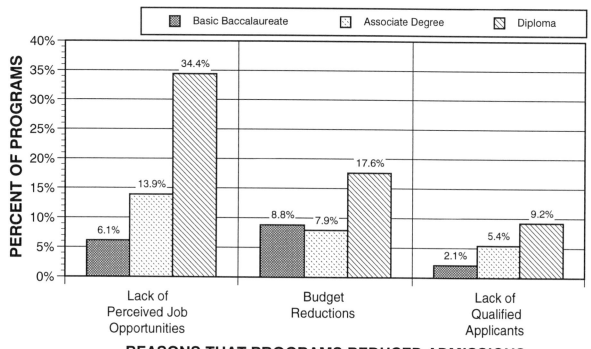

Figure 14
REASONS RN PROGRAMS REDUCED ADMISSIONS

REASONS THAT PROGRAMS REDUCED ADMISSIONS

Section 1-3
Numeric Tables

Table 1
BASIC RN PROGRAMS AND PERCENTAGE CHANGE FROM PREVIOUS YEAR, BY TYPE OF PROGRAM: 1975 TO 1995[1]

YEAR	NUMBER OF SCHOOLS	ALL BASIC RN PROGRAMS		BACCALAUREATE PROGRAMS		ASSOCIATE DEGREE PROGRAMS		DIPLOMA PROGRAMS	
		Number of Programs	Percent Change	Number of Programs	Percent Change	Number of Programs	Percent Change	Number of Programs	Percent Change
1975	1,349	1,362	+0.3	326	+5.2	608	+3.4	428	-7.0
1976	1,337	1,358	-0.3	336	+3.1	632	+3.9	390	-8.9
1977	1,339	1,356	-0.1	344	+2.4	645	+2.1	367	-5.9
1978	1,340	1,358	+0.1	348	+1.2	666	+3.3	344	-6.3
1979	1,354	1,374	+1.2	363	+4.3	678	+1.8	333	-3.2
1980	1,360	1,385	+0.8	377	+3.9	697	+2.8	311	-6.6
1981	1,377	1,401	+1.2	383	+1.6	715	+2.6	303	-2.6
1982	1,406	1,432	+2.2	402	+5.0	742	+3.8	288	-5.0
1983	1,432	1,466	+2.4	421	+4.7	764	+3.0	281	-2.4
1984	1,445	1,477	+0.8	427	+1.4	777	+1.7	273	-2.8
1985	1,434	1,473	-0.2	441	+3.3	776	-0.1	256	-6.2
1986	1,426	1,469	-0.3	455	+3.2	776	-0.0	238	-7.0
1987	1,406	1,465	-0.3	467	+2.6	789	+1.7	209	-12.2
1988	1,391	1,442	-1.6	479	+2.6	792	+0.3	171	-18.7
1989	1,429	1,457	+1.0	488	+1.9	812	+2.5	157	-8.2
1990	1,412	1,470	+0.9	489	+0.2	829	+2.1	152	-3.2
1991	1,411	1,484	+1.0	501	+2.4	838	+1.1	145	-4.6
1992	1,404	1,484	+0.0	501	+0.0	848	+1.2	135	-6.9
1993	1,415[2]	1,493	+0.6	507	+1.2	857	+1.1	129	-4.4
1994	1,422	1,501	+0.5	509	+0.4	868	+1.3	124	-3.9
1995	1,434	1,516	+1.0	521	+2.4	876	+0.9	119	-4.0

[1] Excludes American Samoa, Guam, Puerto Rico, and the Virgin Islands.
[2] Updated information.

Table 2
PUBLIC AND PRIVATE BASIC RN PROGRAMS, BY TYPE OF PROGRAM: 1986 TO 1995[1]

PUBLIC AND PRIVATE NURSING PROGRAMS	NUMBER OF PROGRAMS									
	1986	1987	1988	1989	1990	1991	1992	1993	1994	1995
All Programs	**1,469**	**1,465**	**1,442**	**1,457**	**1,470**	**1,484**	**1,484**	**1,493**	**1,501**	**1,516**
Public	950	970	979	1,005	1,020	1.038	1,036	1,048	1,056	1,052
Private	519	495	463	452	450	446	448	445	445	464
Baccalaureate	455	467	479	488	489	501	501	507	509	521
Public	227	235	239	245	248	254	254	260	265	269
Private	228	232	240	243	241	247	247	247	244	252
Associate Degree	776	789	792	812	829	838	848	857	868	876
Public	688	698	704	726	741	750	754	758	764	766
Private	88	91	88	86	88	88	94	99	104	110
Diploma	238	209	171	157	152	145	135	129	124	119
Public	35	37	36	34	31	34	28	30	27	17
Private	203	172	135	123	121	111	107	99	97	102

[1] Excludes American Samoa, Guam, Puerto Rico, and the Virgin Islands.

Table 3
ALL BASIC RN PROGRAMS, BY NLN REGION AND STATE: 1986 TO 1995[1]

NLN REGION AND STATE	NUMBER OF PROGRAMS									
	1986	1987	1988	1989	1990	1991	1992	1993	1994	1995
United States	**1,469**	**1,465**	**1,442**	**1,457**	**1,470**	**1,484**	**1,484**	**1,493**	**1,501**	**1,516**
North Atlantic	359	355	343	335	331	335	332	329	329	331
Midwest	429	424	415	423	429	430	429	435	434	441
South	478	481	475	483	489	497	500	507	513	516
West	203	205	209	216	221	222	223	222	225	228
Alabama	36	35	35	35	34	33	34	34	36	36
Alaska	2	2	2	3	2	2	2	2	2	2
Arizona	15	15	15	15	15	15	16	16	16	17
Arkansas	20	21	21	21	21	23	24	24	22	22
California	90	89	90	91	91	92	93	93	94	96
Colorado	13	12	12	12	17	17	17	17	17	17
Connecticut	18	18	18	18	18	19	17	17	17	17
Delaware	6	6	6	7	7	7	7	7	7	7
District of Columbia	6	6	5	5	5	5	5	5	5	5
Florida	40	40	40	40	39	39	40	40	40	40
Georgia	34	33	32	33	32	33	32	32	32	33
Hawaii	6	6	6	7	7	7	6	7	7	7
Idaho	6	7	7	7	7	7	7	7	7	8
Illinois	77	72	72	70	69	69	67	70	71	73
Indiana	36	40	42	44	46	44	46	46	46	46
Iowa	39	36	36	37	40	40	40	40	40	42
Kansas	30	32	33	32	32	32	30	30	30	30
Kentucky	28	27	27	29	32	32	33	34	34	35
Louisiana	22	22	21	21	23	23	21	22	23	23
Maine	14	15	15	14	14	14	14	15	15	15
Maryland	24	24	23	23	23	24	24	24	24	23
Massachusetts	46	48	44	41	42	43	42	42	43	44
Michigan	50	49	48	49	50	50	49	50	50	49
Minnesota	25	23	23	20	20	21	21	21	21	21
Mississippi	21	21	21	21	21	21	21	23	23	23
Missouri	41	42	40	44	45	47	46	47	46	48
Montana	6	4	4	5	5	5	5	5	5	5
Nebraska	13	13	10	13	15	13	13	13	13	14
Nevada	5	7	7	6	6	6	6	6	6	6
New Hampshire	10	10	10	9	9	9	9	9	9	9
New Jersey	38	38	38	38	39	38	38	37	37	38
New Mexico	13	13	14	14	14	14	14	14	16	15
New York	110	108	103	101	99	101	103	100	100	100
North Carolina	56	57	57	59	61	62	62	62	62	62
North Dakota	9	8	6	7	6	7	7	7	7	7
Ohio	69	70	67	68	67	68	69	70	69	69
Oklahoma	27	27	27	27	27	27	27	28	28	28
Oregon	17	17	18	18	18	18	18	16	16	16
Pennsylvania	98	94	92	90	87	88	86	86	84	84
Rhode Island	7	7	7	7	6	6	6	6	7	7
South Carolina	19	20	20	20	20	21	20	20	20	21
South Dakota	8	9	9	10	9	8	10	10	10	10
Tennessee	35	35	35	34	35	35	35	35	36	36
Texas	64	64	64	68	69	70	72	73	77	77
Utah	4	4	4	7	7	7	7	7	7	7
Vermont	5	5	5	5	5	5	5	5	5	5
Virginia	35	35	34	34	34	35	36	37	37	37
Washington	23	23	24	24	24	24	24	24	24	24
West Virginia	18	20	18	18	18	19	19	19	19	20
Wisconsin	32	30	29	29	30	31	31	31	31	32
Wyoming	5	6	6	7	8	8	8	8	8	8
American Samoa	1	1	1	1	1	1	1	1	1	1
Guam	1	1	1	1	1	1	1	1	1	1
Puerto Rico	20	20	22	22	22	25	28	29	31	31
Virgin Islands	2	2	2	2	2	2	2	2	2	2

[1] National and regional totals exclude American Samoa, Guam, Puerto Rico, and the Virgin Islands.

Table 4
BASIC BACCALAUREATE NURSING PROGRAMS, BY NLN REGION AND STATE: 1986 TO 1995[1]

NLN REGION AND STATE	NUMBER OF PROGRAMS									
	1986	1987	1988	1989	1990	1991	1992	1993	1994	1995
United States	**455**	**467**	**479**	**488**	**489**	**501**	**501**	**507**	**509**	**521**
North Atlantic	109	110	111	110	109	111	111	113	113	115
Midwest	139	144	151	157	157	161	159	161	160	164
South	154	158	162	165	165	170	172	175	177	181
West	53	55	55	56	58	59	59	58	59	61
Alabama	13	13	13	13	12	12	12	12	12	13
Alaska	1	1	1	1	1	1	1	1	1	1
Arizona	4	4	4	4	4	4	4	4	4	4
Arkansas	7	7	7	7	7	7	8	9	9	9
California	21	21	21	21	22	23	23	23	23	24
Colorado	6	6	6	6	7	7	7	7	7	7
Connecticut	7	7	7	7	7	7	7	8	8	8
Delaware	2	2	2	2	2	2	2	2	2	2
District of Columbia	5	5	4	4	4	4	4	4	4	4
Florida	13	13	13	13	13	13	13	13	13	13
Georgia	13	12	12	13	12	12	12	12	12	13
Hawaii	2	2	2	2	2	2	2	3	3	3
Idaho	1	2	2	2	2	2	2	2	2	3
Illinois	24	24	26	27	27	28	27	27	27	27
Indiana	13	17	20	21	21	21	21	21	20	20
Iowa	11	11	11	11	12	12	12	12	12	12
Kansas	10	11	11	10	10	10	10	11	11	11
Kentucky	9	9	9	10	10	10	10	10	10	10
Louisiana	12	12	12	12	12	12	12	13	13	13
Maine	3	5	6	6	6	6	6	7	7	7
Maryland	6	6	6	6	6	7	7	7	7	7
Massachusetts	14	15	14	14	14	15	15	15	15	16
Michigan	14	14	14	14	14	14	13	14	14	15
Minnesota	11	11	11	8	8	9	9	9	9	9
Mississippi	7	7	7	7	7	7	7	7	7	7
Missouri	11	11	11	14	14	15	15	15	15	17
Montana	2	2	2	2	2	2	2	2	2	2
Nebraska	7	7	7	7	7	6	6	6	6	6
Nevada	1	2	2	2	2	2	2	2	2	2
New Hampshire	3	3	3	3	3	3	3	3	3	3
New Jersey	7	7	7	7	7	7	7	7	7	8
New Mexico	1	1	1	1	1	1	1	1	2	2
New York	33	32	33	32	31	32	32	32	32	32
North Carolina	12	12	12	12	12	12	12	12	12	12
North Dakota	4	4	6	7	6	7	7	7	7	7
Ohio	17	18	18	21	21	22	22	22	22	22
Oklahoma	11	11	11	11	11	11	11	11	11	11
Oregon	4	4	4	5	5	5	5	3	3	3
Pennsylvania	30	30	31	31	31	31	31	31	31	31
Rhode Island	3	3	3	3	3	3	3	3	3	3
South Carolina	6	6	7	7	7	7	7	7	7	8
South Dakota	3	3	3	4	4	4	4	4	4	4
Tennessee	11	12	14	14	15	16	16	16	17	18
Texas	20	20	21	22	23	24	25	25	26	26
Utah	3	3	3	3	3	3	3	3	3	3
Vermont	1	1	1	1	1	1	1	1	1	1
Virginia	9	10	10	10	10	11	11	12	12	12
Washington	6	6	6	6	6	6	6	6	6	6
West Virginia	6	8	8	8	8	9	9	9	9	9
Wisconsin	14	13	13	13	13	13	13	13	13	14
Wyoming	1	1	1	1	1	1	1	1	1	1
American Samoa	0	0	0	0	0	0	0	0	0	0
Guam	0	0	1	1	1	1	1	1	1	1
Puerto Rico	12	12	13	13	13	13	13	14	14	14
Virgin Islands	1	1	1	1	1	1	1	1	1	1

[1] National and regional totals exclude American Samoa, Guam, Puerto Rico, and the Virgin Islands.

Table 5
ASSOCIATE DEGREE NURSING PROGRAMS, BY NLN REGION AND STATE: 1986 TO 1995[1]

NLN REGION AND STATE	NUMBER OF PROGRAMS									
	1986	1987	1988	1989	1990	1991	1992	1993	1994	1995
United States	**776**	**789**	**792**	**812**	**829**	**838**	**848**	**857**	**868**	**876**
North Atlantic	144	147	146	148	147	151	152	151	153	153
Midwest	203	209	211	218	227	228	232	238	241	246
South	281	284	282	287	293	297	301	305	309	311
West	148	149	153	159	162	162	163	163	165	166
Alabama	20	20	20	20	20	20	21	21	23	23
Alaska	1	1	1	2	1	1	1	1	1	1
Arizona	11	11	11	11	11	11	12	12	12	13
Arkansas	11	12	12	12	12	14	14	13	11	11
California	68	67	68	69	68	68	69	69	70	71
Colorado	6	6	6	6	10	10	10	10	10	10
Connecticut	6	6	6	6	6	7	7	6	6	6
Delaware	3	3	3	4	4	4	4	4	4	4
District of Columbia	1	1	1	4	1	1	1	1	1	1
Florida	26	26	26	26	25	25	26	26	26	26
Georgia	19	19	19	19	19	20	20	20	20	20
Hawaii	4	4	4	5	5	5	4	4	4	4
Idaho	5	5	5	5	5	5	5	5	5	5
Illinois	34	34	35	35	35	35	35	38	39	42
Indiana	17	17	19	20	23	22	24	24	25	25
Iowa	20	20	20	21	23	23	23	23	23	25
Kansas	17	19	20	21	21	21	19	19	19	19
Kentucky	19	18	18	19	22	22	23	24	24	25
Louisiana	6	6	6	6	8	8	8	8	9	9
Maine	9	9	9	8	8	8	8	8	8	8
Maryland	14	14	14	14	14	14	14	14	14	14
Massachusetts	19	20	19	19	20	20	20	20	21	21
Michigan	32	32	31	32	33	33	33	33	33	32
Minnesota	12	12	12	12	12	12	12	12	12	12
Mississippi	14	14	14	14	14	14	14	16	16	16
Missouri	20	22	21	22	23	24	25	26	27	27
Montana	2	2	2	3	3	3	3	3	3	3
Nebraska	1	1	2	5	7	6	6	6	6	7
Nevada	4	5	5	4	4	4	4	4	4	4
New Hampshire	6	6	6	6	6	6	6	6	6	6
New Jersey	13	14	14	14	15	14	14	14	14	14
New Mexico	12	12	13	13	13	13	13	13	14	13
New York	59	60	59	60	59	61	63	63	63	63
North Carolina	39	41	41	43	45	46	46	46	46	47
North Dakota	2	2	0	0	0	0	0	0	0	0
Ohio	29	30	31	30	30	31	32	34	34	34
Oklahoma	16	16	16	16	16	16	16	17	17	17
Oregon	13	13	14	13	13	13	13	13	13	13
Pennsylvania	22	22	23	24	22	24	23	23	23	23
Rhode Island	2	2	2	2	2	2	2	2	3	3
South Carolina	12	13	13	13	13	14	13	13	13	13
South Dakota	4	5	5	5	4	4	6	6	6	6
Tennessee	17	17	17	16	16	15	15	15	15	14
Texas	42	42	41	44	44	44	45	46	49	49
Utah	1	1	1	4	4	4	4	4	4	4
Vermont	4	4	4	4	4	4	4	4	4	4
Virginia	16	16	16	16	16	16	17	17	17	17
Washington	17	17	18	18	18	18	18	18	18	18
West Virginia	10	10	9	9	9	9	9	9	9	10
Wisconsin	15	15	15	15	16	17	17	17	17	17
Wyoming	4	5	5	6	7	7	7	7	7	7
American Samoa	1	1	1	1	1	1	1	1	1	1
Guam	1	1	0	0	0	0	0	0	0	0
Puerto Rico	8	8	9	9	9	12	15	15	17	17
Virgin Islands	1	1	1	1	1	1	1	1	1	1

[1] National and regional totals exclude American Samoa, Guam, Puerto Rico, and the Virgin Islands.

Table 6
DIPLOMA NURSING PROGRAMS, BY NLN REGION AND STATE: 1986 TO 1995[1]

NLN REGION AND STATE	NUMBER OF PROGRAMS									
	1986	1987	1988	1989	1990	1991	1992	1993	1994	1995
United States	**238**	**209**	**171**	**157**	**152**	**145**	**135**	**129**	**124**	**119**
North Atlantic	106	98	86	77	75	73	69	65	63	63
Midwest	87	71	53	48	45	41	38	36	33	31
South	43	39	31	31	31	30	27	27	27	24
West	2	1	1	1	1	1	1	1	1	1
Alabama	3	2	2	2	2	1	1	1	1	0
Alaska	0	0	0	0	0	0	0	0	0	0
Arizona	0	0	0	0	0	0	0	0	0	0
Arkansas	2	2	2	2	2	2	2	2	2	2
California	1	1	1	1	1	1	1	1	1	1
Colorado	1	0	0	0	0	0	0	0	0	0
Connecticut	5	5	5	5	5	5	3	3	3	3
Delaware	1	1	1	1	1	1	1	1	1	1
District of Columbia	0	0	0	0	0	0	0	0	0	0
Florida	1	1	1	1	1	1	1	1	1	1
Georgia	2	2	1	1	1	1	0	0	0	0
Hawaii	0	0	0	0	0	0	0	0	0	0
Idaho	0	0	0	0	0	0	0	0	0	0
Illinois	19	14	11	8	7	6	5	5	5	4
Indiana	6	6	3	3	2	1	1	1	1	1
Iowa	8	5	5	5	5	5	5	5	5	5
Kansas	3	2	2	1	1	1	1	0	0	0
Kentucky	0	0	0	0	0	0	0	0	0	0
Louisiana	4	4	3	3	3	3	1	1	1	1
Maine	2	1	0	0	0	0	0	0	0	0
Maryland	4	4	3	3	3	3	3	3	3	2
Massachusetts	13	13	11	8	8	8	7	7	7	7
Michigan	4	3	3	3	3	3	3	3	3	2
Minnesota	2	0	0	0	0	0	0	0	0	0
Mississippi	0	0	0	0	0	0	0	0	0	0
Missouri	10	9	8	8	8	8	6	6	4	4
Montana	0	0	0	0	0	0	0	0	0	0
Nebraska	5	5	1	1	1	1	1	1	1	1
Nevada	0	0	0	0	0	0	0	0	0	0
New Hampshire	1	1	1	0	0	0	0	0	0	0
New Jersey	18	17	17	17	17	17	17	16	16	16
New Mexico	0	0	0	0	0	0	0	0	0	0
New York	18	16	11	9	9	8	8	5	5	5
North Carolina	5	4	4	4	4	4	4	4	4	3
North Dakota	3	2	0	0	0	0	0	0	0	0
Ohio	23	22	18	17	16	15	15	14	13	13
Oklahoma	0	0	0	0	0	0	0	0	0	0
Oregon	0	0	0	0	0	0	0	0	0	0
Pennsylvania	46	42	38	35	34	33	32	32	30	30
Rhode Island	2	2	2	2	1	1	1	1	1	1
South Carolina	1	1	0	0	0	0	0	0	0	0
South Dakota	1	1	1	1	1	0	0	0	0	0
Tennessee	7	6	4	4	4	4	4	4	4	4
Texas	2	2	2	2	2	2	2	2	2	2
Utah	0	0	0	0	0	0	0	0	0	0
Vermont	0	0	0	0	0	0	0	0	0	0
Virginia	10	9	8	8	8	8	8	8	8	8
Washington	0	0	0	0	0	0	0	0	0	0
West Virginia	2	2	1	1	1	1	1	1	1	1
Wisconsin	3	2	1	1	1	1	1	1	1	1
Wyoming	0	0	0	0	0	0	0	0	0	0
American Samoa	0	0	0	0	0	0	0	0	0	0
Guam	0	0	0	0	0	0	0	0	0	0
Puerto Rico	0	0	0	0	0	0	0	0	0	0
Virgin Islands	0	0	0	0	0	0	0	0	0	0

[1] National and regional totals exclude American Samoa, Guam, Puerto Rico, and the Virgin Islands.

Table 7
BACCALAUREATE NURSING PROGRAMS THAT ENROLL BASIC AND/OR RN STUDENTS
BY NLN ACCREDITATION STATUS: JANUARY, 1996[1]

NLN ACCREDITATION STATUS	TOTAL NUMBER OF PROGRAMS	TYPE OF STUDENT ENROLLED	
		Both Basic and RN Students	RN Students Only
Total	**665**	**521**	**144**
Accredited	617	496	121
Non-Accredited	48	25	23

[1] Excludes American Samoa, Guam, Puerto Rico, and the Virgin Islands.

Table 8
Table 8
BASIC RN PROGRAMS, BY TYPE OF PROGRAM AND NLN ACCREDITATION STATUS: JANUARY, 1996[1]

NLN REGION AND STATE	ALL BASIC RN PROGRAMS			BACCALAUREATE PROGRAMS			ASSOCIATE DEGREE PROGRAMS			DIPLOMA PROGRAMS		
	Total	Accredited	Not Accredited	Total	Accredited	Not Accredited	Total	Accredited	Not Accredited	Total	Accredited	Not Accredited
United States	**1,516**	**1,221**	**295**	**521**	**496**	**25**	**876**	**606**	**270**	**119**	**119**	**0**
North Atlantic	331	301	30	115	113	2	153	125	28	63	63	0
Midwest	441	343	98	164	154	10	246	158	88	31	31	0
South	516	414	102	181	170	11	311	220	91	24	24	0
West	228	163	65	61	59	2	166	103	63	1	1	0
Alabama	36	32	4	13	12	1	23	20	3	0	0	0
Alaska	2	2	0	1	1	0	1	1	0	0	0	0
Arizona	17	14	3	4	4	0	13	10	3	0	0	0
Arkansas	22	20	2	9	8	1	11	10	1	2	2	0
California	96	54	42	24	24	0	71	29	42	1	1	0
Colorado	17	10	7	7	6	1	10	4	6	0	0	0
Connecticut	17	16	1	8	7	1	6	6	0	3	3	0
Delaware	7	5	2	2	2	0	4	2	2	1	1	0
District of Columbia	5	5	0	4	4	0	1	1	0	0	0	0
Florida	40	27	13	13	11	2	26	15	11	1	1	0
Georgia	33	32	1	13	12	1	20	20	0	0	0	0
Hawaii	7	5	2	3	2	1	4	3	1	0	0	0
Idaho	8	8	0	3	3	0	5	5	0	0	0	0
Illinois	73	49	24	27	23	4	42	22	20	4	4	0
Indiana	46	40	6	20	20	0	25	19	6	1	1	0
Iowa	42	24	18	12	12	0	25	7	18	5	5	0
Kansas	30	29	1	11	10	1	19	19	0	0	0	0
Kentucky	35	26	9	10	10	0	25	16	9	0	0	0
Louisiana	23	21	2	13	13	0	9	7	2	1	1	0
Maine	15	15	0	7	7	0	8	8	0	0	0	0
Maryland	23	18	5	7	7	0	14	9	5	2	2	0
Massachusetts	44	42	2	16	16	0	21	19	2	7	7	0
Michigan	49	26	23	15	14	1	32	10	22	2	2	0
Minnesota	21	17	4	9	9	0	12	8	4	0	0	0
Mississippi	23	21	2	7	7	0	16	14	2	0	0	0
Missouri	48	36	12	17	16	1	27	16	11	4	4	0
Montana	5	5	0	2	2	0	3	3	0	0	0	0
Nebraska	14	12	2	6	6	0	7	5	2	1	1	0
Nevada	6	6	0	2	2	0	4	4	0	0	0	0
New Hampshire	9	7	2	3	3	0	6	4	2	0	0	0
New Jersey	38	37	1	8	7	1	14	14	0	16	16	0
New Mexico	15	12	3	2	2	0	13	10	3	0	0	0
New York	100	82	18	32	32	0	63	45	18	5	5	0
North Carolina	62	24	38	12	12	0	47	9	38	3	3	0
North Dakota	7	7	0	7	7	0	0	0	0	0	0	0
Ohio	69	64	5	22	20	2	34	31	3	13	13	0
Oklahoma	28	27	1	11	11	0	17	16	1	0	0	0
Oregon	16	11	5	3	3	0	13	8	5	0	0	0
Pennsylvania	84	81	3	31	31	0	23	20	3	30	30	0
Rhode Island	7	6	1	3	3	0	3	2	1	1	1	0
South Carolina	21	16	5	8	6	2	13	10	3	0	0	0
South Dakota	10	8	2	4	4	0	6	4	2	0	0	0
Tennessee	36	34	2	18	16	2	14	14	0	4	4	0
Texas	77	61	16	26	24	2	49	35	14	2	2	0
Utah	7	7	0	3	3	0	4	4	0	0	0	0
Vermont	5	5	0	1	1	0	4	4	0	0	0	0
Virginia	37	36	1	12	12	0	17	16	1	8	8	0
Washington	24	21	3	6	6	0	18	15	3	0	0	0
West Virginia	20	19	1	9	9	0	10	9	1	1	1	0
Wisconsin	32	31	1	14	13	1	17	17	0	1	1	0
Wyoming	8	8	0	1	1	0	7	7	0	0	0	0
American Samoa	1	0	1	0	0	0	1	0	1	0	0	0
Guam	1	0	1	1	0	1	0	0	0	0	0	0
Puerto Rico	31	12	19	14	7	7	17	5	12	0	0	0
Virgin Islands	2	2	0	1	1	0	1	1	0	0	0	0

[1] National and regional totals exclude American Samoa, Guam, Puerto Rico, and the Virgin Islands.

Table 9
MEAN ANNUAL TUITIONS OF FULL-TIME STUDENTS IN PUBLIC OR PRIVATE BASIC RN PROGRAMS: 1995 TO 1996[1]

NURSING PROGRAMS	PRINCIPAL FINANCIAL SUPPORT OF SCHOOL		
	Public		Private
	Resident	Non-Resident	
All Programs	$1,984	$4,973	$7,970
Basic Baccalaureate	$2,903	$7,219	$10,165
Associate Degree	$1,620	$4,141	$7,000
Diploma	$3,379	$4,074	$3,919

[1] Excludes American Samoa, Guam, Puerto Rico, and the Virgin Islands.

Table 10
FALL ADMISSIONS TO PUBLIC AND PRIVATE BASIC RN PROGRAMS, BY TYPE OF PROGRAM: 1986 TO 1995[1]

PUBLIC AND PRIVATE NURSING PROGRAMS	NUMBER OF FALL ADMISSIONS									
	1986	1987	1988	1989	1990	1991	1992	1993	1994	1995
All Programs	**70,581**	**68,745**	**74,921**	**79,570**	**86,125**	**90,499**	**96,786**	**96,864**	**96,107**	**88,901**
Public	50,417	51,362	56,922	60,032	64,410	67,163	70,106	70,216	69,761	64,815
Private	20,164	17,383	17,999	19,538	21,715	23,336	26,680	26,648	26,346	24,086
Baccalaureate	23,765	19,985	20,749	21,544	25,117	27,361	31,719	32,403	33,124	30,186
Public	13,356	12,806	13,122	13,574	15,648	16,369	18,064	18,542	18,422	17,388
Private	10,409	7,179	7,627	7,970	9,469	10,992	13,655	13,861	14,702	12,798
Associate Degree	40,166	41,695	46,910	49,930	52,674	54,732	56,828	56,514	56,035	53,664
Public	36,070	37,389	42,357	44,840	47,175	49,124	50,777	50,170	50,200	46,998
Private	4,096	4,306	4,553	5,090	5,499	5,608	6,051	6,344	5,835	6,666
Diploma	6,650	7,065	7,262	8,096	8,334	8,406	8,239	7,947	6,948	5,051
Public	991	1,167	1,443	1,618	1,587	1,670	1,265	1,504	1,139	429
Private	5,659	5,898	5,819	6,478	6,747	6,736	6,974	6,443	5,809	4,622

[1] Excludes American Samoa, Guam, Puerto Rico, and the Virgin Islands.

Table 11
ANNUAL ADMISSIONS TO BASIC RN PROGRAMS AND PERCENTAGE CHANGE
FROM PREVIOUS YEAR, BY TYPE OF PROGRAM: 1975-76 TO 1994-95[1]

ACADEMIC YEAR	ALL BASIC RN PROGRAMS		BACCALAUREATE PROGRAMS		ASSOCIATE DEGREE PROGRAMS		DIPLOMA PROGRAMS	
	Number of Admissions	Percent Change	Number of Admissions	Percent Change	Number of Admissions	Percent Change	Number of Admissions	Percent Change
1975-76	112,174	+2.9	36,320	+3.9	52,232	+5.8	23,622	-4.3
1976-77	112,523	+0.3	36,670	+1.0	53,610	+2.6	22,243	-5.8
1977-78	110,950	-1.4	37,348	+1.8	52,991	-1.1	20,611	-7.3
1978-79	107,476	-3.2	35,611	-4.7	53,366	+0.7	18,499	-10.2
1979-80	105,952	-1.4	35,414	-0.5	53,633	+0.5	16,905	-8.6
1980-81	110,201	+4.0	35,808	+1.1	56,899	+6.1	17,494	+3.5
1981-82	115,279	+4.6	35,928	+0.3	60,423	+6.1	18,928	+8.1
1982-83	120,579	+4.6	37,264	+3.7	63,947	+5.8	19,368	+2.3
1983-84	123,824	+2.7	39,400	+5.7	66,576	+4.1	17,848	-7.8
1984-85	118,224	-4.5	39,573	+0.4	63,776	-4.2	14,875	-16.7
1985-86	100,791	-14.7	34,310	-13.3	56,635	-11.2	9,846	-33.0
1986-87	90,693	-10.0	28,026	-18.3	54,330	-4.1	8,337	-15.3
1987-88	94,269	+3.9	28,505	+1.7	57,375	+5.6	8,389	+0.6
1988-89	103,025	+9.3	29,042	+1.9	63,973	+11.5	10,010	+19.3
1989-90	108,580	+5.4	29,858	+2.6	68,634	+7.3	10,088	+0.8
1990-91	113,526	+4.6	33,437	+12.0	69,869	+1.8	10,220	-1.3
1991-92	122,656	+8.0	37,886	+13.3	74,079	+6.0	10,691	+4.6
1992-93	126,837	+3.4	41,290	+9.0	75,382	+1.7	10,165	-4.9
1993-94	129,897	+2.4	42,953	+4.0	77,343	+2.6	9,601	-5.5
1994-95	127,184	-2.1	43,451	+1.2	76,016	-1.7	7,717	-19.6

[1] Excludes American Samoa, Guam, Puerto Rico, and the Virgin Islands.

Table 12
ANNUAL ADMISSIONS TO PUBLIC AND PRIVATE BASIC RN PROGRAMS, BY TYPE OF PROGRAM: 1985-86 TO 1994-95[1]

PUBLIC AND PRIVATE NURSING PROGRAMS	NUMBER OF ANNUAL ADMISSIONS									
	1985-86	1986-87	1987-88	1988-89	1989-90	1990-91	1991-92	1992-93	1993-94	1994-95
All Programs	**100,791**	**90,693**	**94,269**	**103,025**	**108,580**	**113,526**	**122,656**	**126,837**	**129,897**	**127,184**
Public	71,921	67,890	71,866	77,892	82,686	88,764	92,720	94,572	96,296	89,819
Private	28,870	22,803	22,403	25,133	25,894	24,762	29,936	32,265	33,601	37,365
Baccalaureate	34,310	28,026	28,505	29,042	29,858	33,437	37,886	41,290	42,953	43,451
Public	19,747	18,057	18,622	18,824	19,492	22,252	23,484	24,345	24,861	24,909
Private	14,563	9,969	9,883	10,218	10,366	11,185	14,402	16,945	18,092	18,542
Associate Degree	56,635	54,330	57,375	63,973	68,634	69,869	74,079	75,382	77,343	76,016
Public	50,549	48,249	51,566	56,958	61,151	64,258	67,146	68,075	69,562	64,012
Private	6,086	6,081	5,809	7,015	7,483	5,611	6,933	7,307	7,781	12,004
Diploma	9,846	8,337	8,389	10,010	10,088	10,220	10,691	10,165	9,601	7,717
Public	1,625	1,584	1,678	2,110	2,043	2,254	2,090	2,152	1,873	898
Private	8,221	6,753	6,711	7,900	8,045	7,966	8,601	8,013	7,728	6,819

[1] Excludes American Samoa, Guam, Puerto Rico, and the Virgin Islands.

Table 13
ANNUAL ADMISSIONS TO ALL BASIC RN PROGRAMS, BY NLN REGION AND STATE: 1985-86 TO 1994-95[1]

NLN REGION AND STATE	NUMBER OF ADMISSIONS									
	1985-86	1986-87	1987-88	1988-89	1989-90	1990-91	1991-92	1992-93	1993-94	1994-95
United States	**100,791**	**90,693**	**94,269**	**103,025**	**108,580**	**113,526**	**122,656**	**126,837**	**129,897**	**127,184**
North Atlantic	27,818	23,069	23,792	25,876	26,889	27,349	30,556	32,589	33,140	32,757
Midwest	27,305	25,151	24,647	26,862	28,410	29,602	32,527	33,579	34,840	34,225
South	31,702	29,632	32,380	36,083	39,397	42,468	45,062	45,764	46,979	45,311
West	13,966	12,841	13,450	14,204	13,884	14,107	14,511	14,905	14,938	14,891
Alabama	2,158	2,149	2,003	2,346	2,574	2,570	3,108	3,488	3,847	3,718
Alaska	171	166	166	266	81	103	102	105	110	108
Arizona	1,024	962	970	996	929	1,110	1,196	1,237	1,281	1,369
Arkansas	937	983	1,327	1,415	1,545	1,723	1,821	1,802	1,751	1,500
California	7,013	6,098	6,320	6,507	6,340	6,465	6,577	6,691	6,710	6,998
Colorado	787	942	873	1,092	926	1,011	1,020	1,064	1,041	1,098
Connecticut	1,266	1,012	1,200	1,200	1,070	1,141	1,513	1,370	1,049	1,291
Delaware	413	339	370	386	394	316	455	580	532	561
District of Columbia	627	334	449	315	248	361	327	555	355	373
Florida	3,508	3,426	3,651	3,849	4,400	4,551	4,688	4,930	4,835	5,173
Georgia	2,060	1,805	2,075	2,289	2,725	2,566	3,003	3,252	3,366	3,298
Hawaii	372	183	345	272	361	281	301	409	395	337
Idaho	303	274	391	332	338	372	331	333	352	330
Illinois	5,255	4,422	3,840	4,642	4,453	4,889	5,284	5,317	5,774	6,316
Indiana	2,551	2,480	2,496	2,581	2,594	2,820	3,038	3,213	3,257	3,404
Iowa	1,625	1,661	1,668	1,672	1,852	1,938	2,146	2,418	2,358	2,279
Kansas	1,131	957	1,165	1,244	1,613	1,521	1,610	1,831	1,603	1,565
Kentucky	2,236	1,683	1,879	2,093	2,159	3,048	2,729	2,676	2,757	2,596
Louisiana	1,768	1,432	1,558	1,741	2,081	3,100	2,970	2,813	3,156	2,984
Maine	490	433	421	514	498	579	490	797	602	820
Maryland	1,788	1,483	1,449	1,542	1,566	1,819	2,166	2,268	2,269	2,070
Massachusetts	3,065	2,700	2,545	2,536	3,082	3,020	3,415	3,422	3,386	3,277
Michigan	3,893	3,872	3,521	3,582	3,748	3,890	4,308	4,139	4,236	4,120
Minnesota	1,343	1,431	1,570	1,788	1,939	1,759	1,974	2,042	1,997	1,915
Mississippi	1,524	1,503	1,440	1,584	1,988	2,089	2,144	2,184	2,211	2,117
Missouri	2,081	2,087	1,962	2,196	2,350	2,535	3,049	2,999	3,380	3,572
Montana	305	284	322	347	334	366	368	355	387	369
Nebraska	567	749	663	845	978	859	891	960	1,051	1,000
Nevada	204	199	268	215	256	281	268	283	319	300
New Hampshire	412	372	422	360	538	504	551	579	543	615
New Jersey	3,275	2,521	2,890	3,198	2,913	3,426	3,794	3,574	3,631	3,173
New Mexico	421	455	731	713	788	778	798	710	824	705
New York	11,845	9,401	9,122	10,638	10,861	10,735	11,678	12,571	13,942	14,570
North Carolina	2,796	2,920	2,881	3,526	3,753	3,599	3,597	3,833	4,141	3,817
North Dakot	327	225	191	301	374	341	381	320	406	312
Ohio	5,203	4,767	4,960	5,386	5,824	6,086	6,232	6,771	7,374	6,367
Oklahoma	1,232	1,244	1,335	1,350	1,513	1,642	1,761	1,657	1,710	1,712
Oregon	924	953	875	963	975	968	1,017	981	938	838
Pennsylvania	5,742	5,335	5,758	6,100	6,564	6,421	7,136	7,934	8,142	7,173
Rhode Island	522	440	402	382	486	579	886	902	673	662
South Carolina	1,231	1,031	1,239	1,387	1,579	1,763	1,742	1,673	1,778	1,703
South Dakota	361	629	542	365	486	473	561	579	554	535
Tennessee	2,341	2,179	2,848	2,702	3,025	2,940	3,191	3,440	3,654	3,250
Texas	5,053	4,758	5,631	6,880	6,905	7,273	7,851	7,533	7,344	7,282
Utah	473	345	450	507	810	523	680	719	685	666
Vermont	211	182	213	247	235	267	311	305	285	242
Virginia	2,024	2,035	2,149	2,597	2,551	2,665	3,151	3,030	3,027	2,975
Washington	1,751	1,769	1,544	1,770	1,547	1,552	1,527	1,704	1,626	1,486
West Virginia	1,046	1,001	915	1,052	1,033	1,120	1,140	1,185	1,133	1,116
Wisconsin	2,968	1,871	2,069	2,278	2,199	2,491	3,053	2,990	2,850	2,840
Wyoming	168	211	195	224	199	297	326	314	270	287
American Samoa	34	11	11	11	11	10	11	12	12	10
Guam	29	29	0	25	20	25	25	19	20	25
Puerto Rico	3,263	3,048	1,945	1,729	1,816	1,507	1,398	1,859	1,570	2,057
Virgin Islands	28	36	19	12	19	20	27	40	65	80

[1] National and regional totals exclude American Samoa, Guam, Puerto Rico, and the Virgin Islands.

Table 14
ANNUAL ADMISSIONS TO BASIC BACCALAUREATE NURSING PROGRAMS, BY NLN REGION AND STATE: 1985-86 TO 1994-95[1]

NLN REGION AND STATE	NUMBER OF ADMISSIONS									
	1985-86	1986-87	1987-88	1988-89	1989-90	1990-91	1991-92	1992-93	1993-94	1994-95
United States	**34,310**	**28,026**	**28,505**	**29,042**	**29,858**	**33,437**	**37,886**	**41,290**	**42,953**	**43,451**
North Atlantic	9,491	6,545	6,449	6,525	6,412	6,549	7,612	9,845	9,746	9,673
Midwest	9,704	8,394	8,267	8,439	8,614	9,258	11,380	12,391	13,154	13,346
South	10,584	9,064	9,666	9,937	11,145	13,240	14,419	14,475	15,299	15,167
West	4,531	4,023	4,123	4,141	3,687	4,390	4,475	4,579	4,754	5,265
Alabama	861	976	834	853	915	821	1,096	1,086	1,091	1,143
Alaska	132	126	126	226	38	53	65	69	78	80
Arizona	314	279	270	287	191	270	285	337	347	452
Arkansas	258	289	310	321	317	447	426	471	591	478
California	2,083	1,746	1,720	1,595	1,371	1,769	1,802	1,696	1,768	2,298
Colorado	347	398	299	455	350	460	409	477	506	575
Connecticut	374	349	516	574	277	342	656	707	456	650
Delaware	171	117	117	122	88	72	188	278	256	283
District of Columbia	562	255	359	225	199	279	263	491	293	311
Florida	926	714	652	770	779	915	925	1,015	940	1,010
Georgia	725	503	561	769	987	755	940	909	1,016	1,063
Hawaii	147	119	170	59	152	104	101	185	196	143
Idaho	45	44	78	87	69	85	74	90	90	90
Illinois	1,694	1,354	1,162	1,242	1,052	1,341	1,645	1,851	2,278	2,653
Indiana	1,207	1,082	1,116	1,092	995	1,188	1,271	1,362	1,338	1,455
Iowa	451	394	377	354	436	367	467	542	489	512
Kansas	436	353	403	428	523	507	643	899	694	664
Kentucky	977	554	607	662	566	815	738	635	785	811
Louisiana	974	790	911	1,009	1,247	2,184	1,925	1,708	2,086	1,978
Maine	206	205	226	311	283	338	196	426	237	425
Maryland	612	466	388	306	377	554	740	829	762	742
Massachusetts	1,114	823	715	785	1,134	998	1,180	1,190	1,227	1,171
Michigan	1,100	1,177	1,069	1,080	968	1,137	1,232	1,298	1,344	1,304
Minnesota	503	437	445	418	503	475	568	769	688	725
Mississippi	407	362	322	348	570	689	738	665	684	623
Missouri	631	569	601	557	528	702	1,019	967	1,262	1,537
Montana	187	176	220	187	221	239	233	224	258	235
Nebraska	346	608	538	610	648	499	572	617	745	644
Nevada	42	43	71	75	85	118	90	126	114	111
New Hampshire	117	110	81	99	136	151	168	175	162	152
New Jersey	1,027	528	681	408	386	397	459	422	562	478
New Mexico	26	55	77	74	145	227	192	40	128	160
New York	3,669	2,339	1,957	2,115	1,948	1,759	1,765	2,613	2,948	3,157
North Carolina	587	837	553	587	658	808	814	1,038	1,122	1,049
North Dakota	179	162	191	301	374	341	381	320	406	312
Ohio	1,389	1,265	1,219	1,282	1,507	1,447	1,916	2,077	2,272	1,966
Oklahoma	455	372	407	414	447	503	647	536	582	560
Oregon	292	370	288	286	327	369	434	378	376	318
Pennsylvania	2,025	1,611	1,618	1,738	1,724	1,931	2,080	2,903	3,259	2,730
Rhode Island	203	152	104	92	174	204	565	561	266	248
South Carolina	469	282	355	342	326	555	534	527	525	428
South Dakota	143	140	181	125	206	254	281	218	214	221
Tennessee	629	576	1,000	729	908	736	932	1,187	1,213	1,341
Texas	1,698	1,517	1,728	1,732	2,072	2,340	2,832	2,404	2,487	2,528
Utah	212	170	231	203	341	221	270	250	258	269
Vermont	73	56	75	56	63	78	92	79	80	68
Virginia	662	587	753	776	701	789	775	1,037	995	958
Washington	601	419	514	558	397	420	461	643	571	469
West Virginia	344	239	285	319	275	329	357	428	420	455
Wisconsin	1,625	853	965	950	874	1,000	1,385	1,471	1,424	1,353
Wyoming	53	78	59	49	0	55	59	64	64	65
American Samoa	0	0	0	0	0	0	0	0	0	0
Guam	0	0	0	25	20	25	25	19	20	25
Puerto Rico	2,466	2,335	1,301	996	900	672	686	786	804	910
Virgin Islands	10	18	9	7	5	10	18	25	42	52

[1] National and regional totals exclude American Samoa, Guam, Puerto Rico, and the Virgin Islands.

33

Table 15
ANNUAL ADMISSIONS TO ASSOCIATE DEGREE NURSING PROGRAMS,
BY NLN REGION AND STATE: 1985-86 TO 1994-95[1]

NLN REGION AND STATE	NUMBER OF ANNUAL ADMISSIONS									
	1985-86	1986-87	1987-88	1988-89	1989-90	1990-91	1991-92	1992-93	1993-94	1994-95
United States	**56,635**	**54,330**	**57,375**	**63,973**	**68,634**	**69,869**	**74,079**	**75,382**	**77,343**	**76,016**
North Atlantic	14,089	12,800	13,592	14,792	15,970	15,952	17,990	18,018	18,893	19,206
Midwest	14,012	13,974	13,927	15,652	16,888	17,503	18,117	18,369	19,356	18,952
South	19,285	18,894	20,695	23,753	25,816	26,940	28,170	28,864	29,071	28,391
West	9,249	8,662	9,161	9,776	9,960	9,474	9,802	10,131	10,023	9,467
Alabama	1,265	1,139	1,136	1,457	1,632	1,719	1,956	2,348	2,710	2,575
Alaska	39	40	40	40	43	50	37	36	32	28
Arizona	710	683	700	709	738	840	911	900	934	917
Arkansas	576	543	705	767	870	861	954	911	795	773
California	4,744	4,196	4,434	4,625	4,732	4,453	4,541	4,800	4,781	4,541
Colorado	440	544	574	637	576	551	611	587	535	523
Connecticut	712	442	457	356	472	512	672	478	413	467
Delaware	224	205	236	245	276	212	237	272	248	249
District of Columbia	65	79	90	90	49	82	64	64	62	62
Florida	2,513	2,636	2,920	2,980	3,508	3,522	3,656	3,817	3,798	4,074
Georgia	1,233	1,215	1,420	1,432	1,738	1,811	2,063	2,343	2,350	2,235
Hawaii	225	64	175	213	209	177	200	224	199	194
Idaho	258	230	313	245	269	287	257	243	262	240
Illinois	2,847	2,723	2,418	3,024	3,032	3,247	3,342	3,139	3,244	3,459
Indiana	1,041	1,076	1,263	1,389	1,550	1,576	1,689	1,778	1,849	1,921
Iowa	968	1,006	1,124	1,111	1,114	1,237	1,293	1,466	1,582	1,499
Kansas	608	580	733	792	1,062	984	967	932	909	901
Kentucky	1,259	1,129	1,272	1,431	1,593	2,233	1,991	2,041	1,972	1,785
Louisiana	457	438	412	509	618	868	1,003	1,060	1,014	963
Maine	260	228	195	203	215	241	294	371	365	395
Maryland	1,077	899	927	1,079	1,061	1,098	1,220	1,235	1,324	1,265
Massachusetts	1,517	1,479	1,482	1,361	1,492	1,508	1,706	1,680	1,634	1,659
Michigan	2,489	2,451	2,298	2,348	2,584	2,458	2,763	2,586	2,647	2,692
Minnesota	840	994	1,125	1,370	1,436	1,284	1,406	1,273	1,309	1,190
Mississippi	1,117	1,141	1,118	1,236	1,418	1,400	1,406	1,519	1,527	1,494
Missouri	938	1,032	860	1,025	1,149	1,208	1,367	1,530	1,658	1,725
Montana	118	108	102	160	113	127	135	131	129	134
Nebraska	70	83	71	184	267	285	254	258	248	260
Nevada	162	156	197	140	171	163	178	157	205	189
New Hampshire	251	248	341	261	402	353	383	404	381	463
New Jersey	1,267	1,156	1,340	1,415	1,477	1,737	1,752	1,775	1,652	1,595
New Mexico	395	400	654	639	643	551	606	670	696	545
New York	7,521	6,592	6,743	8,013	8,453	8,494	9,496	9,643	10,761	11,116
North Carolina	2,042	1,969	2,150	2,414	2,741	2,501	2,499	2,513	2,666	2,541
North Dakota	89	63	0	0	0	0	0	0	0	0
Ohio	2,689	2,608	2,705	2,968	3,177	3,611	3,237	3,597	4,214	3,574
Oklahoma	777	872	928	936	1,066	1,139	1,114	1,121	1,128	1,152
Oregon	632	583	587	677	648	599	583	603	562	520
Pennsylvania	1,884	1,998	2,309	2,398	2,682	2,294	2,886	2,805	2,813	2,663
Rhode Island	250	247	261	259	280	330	281	300	359	363
South Carolina	749	740	884	1,045	1,253	1,208	1,208	1,146	1,253	1,275
South Dakota	186	385	305	217	280	219	280	361	340	314
Tennessee	1,261	1,301	1,432	1,462	1,630	1,767	1,771	1,675	1,649	1,507
Texas	3,245	3,111	3,764	4,948	4,641	4,725	4,779	4,898	4,625	4,519
Utah	267	175	219	304	469	302	410	469	427	397
Vermont	138	126	138	191	172	189	219	226	205	174
Virginia	1,073	1,150	1,077	1,406	1,374	1,377	1,854	1,566	1,625	1,634
Washington	1,150	1,350	1,030	1212	1,150	1,132	1,066	1,061	1,055	1,017
West Virginia	641	611	550	651	673	711	696	671	635	599
Wisconsin	1,247	973	1,025	1,224	1,237	1,394	1,519	1,449	1,356	1,417
Wyoming	115	133	136	175	199	242	267	250	206	222
American Samoa	34	11	11	11	11	10	11	12	12	10
Guam	29	29	0	0	0	0	0	0	0	0
Puerto Rico	797	713	644	733	916	835	712	1,073	766	1,147
Virgin Islands	18	18	10	5	14	10	9	15	23	28

[1] National and regional totals exclude American Samoa, Guam, Puerto Rico, and the Virgin Islands.

Table 16
ANNUAL ADMISSIONS TO DIPLOMA NURSING PROGRAMS,
BY NLN REGION AND STATE: 1985-86 TO 1994-95[1]

NLN REGION AND STATE	NUMBER OF ANNUAL ADMISSIONS									
	1985-86	1986-87	1987-88	1988-89	1989-90	1990-91	1991-92	1992-93	1993-94	1994-95
United States	**9,846**	**8,337**	**8,389**	**10,010**	**10,088**	**10,220**	**10,691**	**10,165**	**9,601**	**7,717**
North Atlantic	4,238	3,724	3,751	4,559	4,507	4,848	4,954	4,726	4,501	3,878
Midwest	3,589	2,783	2,453	2,771	2,908	2,841	3,030	2,819	2,330	1,927
South	1,833	1,674	2,019	2,393	2,436	2,288	2,473	2,425	2,609	1,753
West	186	156	166	287	237	243	234	195	161	159
Alabama	32	34	33	36	27	30	56	54	46	0
Alaska	0	0	0	0	0	0	0	0	0	0
Arizona	0	0	0	0	0	0	0	0	0	0
Arkansas	103	151	312	327	358	415	441	420	365	249
California	186	156	166	287	237	243	234	195	161	159
Colorado	0	0	0	0	0	0	0	0	0	0
Connecticut	180	221	227	270	321	287	185	185	180	174
Delaware	18	17	17	19	30	32	30	30	28	29
District of Columbia	0	0	0	0	0	0	0	0	0	0
Florida	69	76	79	99	113	114	107	98	97	89
Georgia	102	87	94	88	0	0	0	0	0	0
Hawaii	0	0	0	0	0	0	0	0	0	0
Idaho	0	0	0	0	0	0	0	0	0	0
Illinois	714	345	260	358	369	301	297	327	252	204
Indiana	303	322	117	100	49	56	78	73	70	28
Iowa	206	261	167	207	302	334	386	410	287	268
Kansas	87	24	29	24	28	30	0	0	0	0
Kentucky	0	0	0	0	0	0	0	0	0	0
Louisiana	337	204	235	223	216	48	42	45	56	43
Maine	24	0	0	0	0	0	0	0	0	0
Maryland	99	118	134	157	128	167	206	204	183	63
Massachusetts	434	398	348	390	456	514	529	552	525	447
Michigan	304	244	154	154	196	295	313	255	245	124
Minnesota	0	0	0	0	0	0	0	0	0	0
Mississippi	0	0	0	0	0	0	0	0	0	0
Missouri	512	486	501	614	673	625	663	502	460	310
Montana	0	0	0	0	0	0	0	0	0	0
Nebraska	151	58	54	51	63	75	65	85	58	96
Nevada	0	0	0	0	0	0	0	0	0	0
New Hampshire	44	14	0	0	0	0	0	0	0	0
New Jersey	981	837	869	1,375	1,050	1,292	1,583	1,377	1,417	1,100
New Mexico	0	0	0	0	0	0	0	0	0	0
New York	655	470	422	510	460	482	417	315	233	297
North Carolina	167	114	178	255	354	290	284	282	353	227
North Dakota	59	0	0	0	0	0	0	0	0	0
Ohio	1,125	894	1,036	1,136	1,140	1,028	1,079	1,097	888	827
Oklahoma	0	0	0	0	0	0	0	0	0	0
Oregon	0	0	0	0	0	0	0	0	0	0
Pennsylvania	1,833	1,726	1,831	1,964	2,158	2,196	2,170	2,226	2,070	1,780
Rhode Island	69	41	37	31	32	45	40	41	48	51
South Carolina	13	9	0	0	0	0	0	0	0	0
South Dakota	32	104	56	23	0	0	0	0	0	0
Tennessee	451	302	416	511	487	437	488	578	792	402
Texas	110	130	139	200	192	208	240	231	232	235
Utah	0	0	0	0	0	0	0	0	0	0
Vermont	0	0	0	0	0	0	0	0	0	0
Virginia	289	298	319	415	476	499	522	427	407	383
Washington	0	0	0	0	0	0	0	0	0	0
West Virginia	61	151	80	82	85	80	87	86	78	62
Wisconsin	96	45	79	104	88	97	149	70	70	70
Wyoming	0	0	0	0	0	0	0	0	0	0
American Samoa	0	0	0	0	0	0	0	0	0	0
Guam	0	0	0	0	0	0	0	0	0	0
Puerto Rico	0	0	0	0	0	0	0	0	0	0
Virgin Islands	0	0	0	0	0	0	0	0	0	0

[1] National and regional totals exclude American Samoa, Guam, Puerto Rico, and the Virgin Islands.

Table 17
ENROLLMENTS IN BASIC RN PROGRAMS AND PERCENTAGE CHANGE
FROM PREVIOUS YEAR, BY TYPE OF PROGRAM: 1976 TO 1995[1]

YEAR	ALL BASIC RN PROGRAMS		BACCALAUREATE PROGRAMS		ASSOCIATE DEGREE PROGRAMS		DIPLOMA PROGRAMS	
	Number of Enrollments	Percent Change	Number of Enrollments	Percent Change	Number of Enrollments	Percent Change	Number of Enrollments	Percent Change
1976	247,044	-0.4	99,949	+0.1	91,004	+3.3	56,091	-6.8
1977	245,390	-0.7	101,430	+1.5	91,102	+0.1	52,858	-5.8
1978	239,486	-2.4	99,900	-1.5	91,527	+0.5	48,059	-9.1
1979	234,659	-2.0	98,939	-1.0	92,069	+0.6	43,651	-9.2
1980	230,966	-1.6	95,858	-3.1	94,060	+2.2	41,048	-6.0
1981	234,995	+1.7	93,967	-2.0	100,019	+6.3	41,009	-0.1
1982	242,035	+3.0	94,363	+0.4	105,324	+5.3	42,348	+3.3
1983	250,553	+3.5	98,941	+4.9	109,605	+4.1	42,007	-0.8
1984	237,232	-5.3	95,008	-4.0	104,968	-4.2	37,256	-11.3
1985	217,955	-8.1	91,020	-4.2	96,756	-7.8	30,179	-19.0
1986	193,712	-11.1	81,602	-10.3	89,469	-7.5	22,641	-25.0
1987	182,947	-5.6	73,621	-9.8	90,399	+1.0	18,927	-16.4
1988	184,924	+1.1	70,078	-4.8	95,986	+6.2	18,860	-0.4
1989	201,458	+8.9	74,865	+6.8	106,175	+10.6	20,418	+8.3
1990	221,170	+9.8	81,788	+9.2	117,413	+10.6	21,969	+7.6
1991	237,598	+7.4	90,877	+11.1	123,816	+5.4	22,905	+4.3
1992	257,983	+8.6	102,128	+12.4	132,603	+7.1	23,252	+1.5
1993	270,228	+4.7	110,693	+8.4	137,300	+3.5	22,235	-4.4
1994	268,350	-0.7	112,659	+1.8	135,895	-1.0	19,796	-11.0
1995	261,219	-2.7	109,505	-2.8	135,235	-0.5	16,479	-16.8

[1] Excludes American Samoa, Guam, Puerto Rico, and the Virgin Islands.

Table 18
ENROLLMENTS IN PUBLIC AND PRIVATE BASIC RN PROGRAMS, BY TYPE OF PROGRAM: 1986 TO 1995[1]

PUBLIC AND PRIVATE NURSING PROGRAMS	TOTAL ENROLLMENTS									
	1986	1987	1988	1989	1990	1991	1992	1993	1994	1995
All Programs	**193,715**	**182,947**	**184,924**	**201,458**	**221,170**	**237,598**	**257,983**	**270,228**	**268,350**	**261,219**
Public	129,362	130,230	134,575	148,343	162,707	176,892	186,230	193,951	191,193	176,828
Private	64,350	52,717	50,349	53,115	58,463	60,706	71,753	76,277	77,157	84,391
Baccalaureate	81,602	73,621	70,078	74,865	81,788	90,877	102,128	110,693	112,659	109,505
Public	47,329	47,276	45,414	49,792	54,245	59,257	62,045	65,643	65,331	62,514
Private	34,273	26,345	24,664	25,073	27,543	31,620	40,083	45,050	47,328	46,991
Associate Degree	89,469	90,399	95,986	106,175	117,413	123,816	132,603	137,300	135,895	135,235
Public	78,207	79,542	85,413	94,501	104,311	112,576	120,030	123,794	122,061	112,393
Private	11,262	10,857	10,573	11,674	13,102	11,240	12,573	13,506	13,834	22,842
Diploma	22,641	18,927	18,860	20,418	21,969	22,905	23,252	22,235	19,796	16,479
Public	3,826	3,412	3,748	4,050	4,151	5,059	4,155	4,514	3,801	1,921
Private	18,815	15,515	15,112	16,368	17,818	17,846	19,097	17,721	15,995	14,558

[1] Excludes American Samoa, Guam, Puerto Rico, and the Virgin Islands.

Table 19
TOTAL ENROLLMENTS IN ALL BASIC RN PROGRAMS, BY NLN REGION AND STATE: 1986 TO 1995[1]

NLN REGION AND STATE	NUMBER OF TOTAL ENROLLMENTS									
	1986	1987	1988	1989	1990	1991	1992	1993	1994	1995
United States	**193,712**	**182,947**	**184,924**	**201,458**	**221,170**	**237,598**	**257,983**	**270,228**	**268,350**	**261,219**
North Atlantic	56,345	50,521	49,533	53,315	56,673	60,276	68,512	72,271	74,088	75,344
Midwest	54,591	50,450	49,957	53,665	59,682	64,100	67,540	71,221	71,004	68,464
South	58,316	57,674	60,912	68,882	77,851	84,704	92,796	97,530	94,284	88,982
West	24,460	24,302	24,522	25,596	26,964	28,518	29,135	29,206	28,974	28,429
Alabama	4,300	3,799	4,003	4,462	4,886	5,704	6,962	8,008	8,380	7,637
Alaska	455	268	269	274	268	231	228	224	269	275
Arizona	1,816	1,827	1,819	1,765	1,799	1,881	2,095	2,350	2,309	2,363
Arkansas	1,936	1,929	2,170	2,627	3,268	3,628	3,734	3,534	3,347	2,880
California	11,992	12,108	11,668	12,003	12,455	13,511	13,599	13,526	13,525	13,074
Colorado	1,446	1,393	1,336	1,592	1,706	1,823	1,937	2,096	1,903	1,983
Connecticut	2,551	2,267	2,268	2,371	2,506	2,784	2,734	2,760	2,796	2,777
Delaware	957	829	800	879	937	809	1,155	1,327	1,332	1,228
District of Columbia	1,055	754	799	704	710	759	877	983	1,051	1,141
Florida	5,545	5,475	5,877	6,371	7,181	7,800	8,166	8,510	8,918	8,809
Georgia	3,278	3,185	3,532	3,942	4,450	5,026	5,785	6,259	6,078	5,634
Hawaii	464	520	825	659	624	466	665	824	911	992
Idaho	470	550	625	710	885	722	684	692	704	670
Illinois	9,246	8,087	8,114	8,532	9,171	9,819	10,752	11,522	12,104	12,388
Indiana	6,260	5,830	6,007	6,219	7,916	8,027	6,871	7,093	7,370	7,594
Iowa	2,966	2,917	2,817	3,126	3,420	3,705	4,280	4,519	4,349	4,004
Kansas	1,775	1,791	1,951	2,272	2,721	2,725	3,015	3,125	3,072	2,870
Kentucky	3,521	3,550	3,801	4,250	4,515	5,527	5,914	5,663	5,594	5,177
Louisiana	5,081	4,957	5,462	7,163	7,620	7,604	10,336	12,240	10,130	9,212
Maine	910	1,001	984	1,153	1,350	1,508	1,827	1,969	1,934	1,628
Maryland	3,097	2,775	2,629	2,838	3,055	3,424	4,071	4,015	4,099	3,899
Massachusetts	7,119	6,239	5,593	6,232	6,513	7,062	7,883	8,313	8,334	8,147
Michigan	7,540	7,553	6,928	7,219	7,575	8,270	8,865	8,796	8,977	8,730
Minnesota	2,659	2,548	2,480	2,774	3,018	3,293	3,318	3,521	3,357	3,228
Mississippi	2,669	2,584	2,720	2,980	3,488	3,658	3,974	3,995	3,761	3,623
Missouri	4,218	3,875	3,702	3,943	4,421	5,032	5,956	6,337	6,017	6,018
Montana	887	739	868	896	916	888	994	974	915	885
Nebraska	1,266	1,169	1,196	1,603	2,011	2,369	2,535	2,552	2,458	2,273
Nevada	477	488	439	452	568	638	490	556	513	534
New Hampshire	819	803	805	905	1,116	1,243	1,408	1,422	1,418	1,369
New Jersey	5,942	5,410	5,642	5,959	6,418	7,140	7,788	7,886	7,698	7,079
New Mexico	757	920	987	1,072	1,220	1,337	1,386	1,347	1,428	1,310
New York	21,380	19,266	18,105	19,414	20,056	21,110	24,515	26,656	28,916	33,368
North Carolina	4,600	4,679	5,086	5,852	6,677	6,721	7,000	7,304	7,251	7,135
North Dakota	865	650	551	738	862	722	913	808	777	732
Ohio	11,156	10,651	10,748	11,464	11,866	12,523	13,450	14,218	14,487	13,372
Oklahoma	1,977	2,324	2,243	2,562	2,840	3,241	3,363	3,345	3,251	3,130
Oregon	1,676	1,620	1,595	1,747	1,851	2,012	1,967	1,480	1,680	1,642
Pennsylvania	13,832	12,325	13,106	14,159	15,294	15,776	18,069	18,596	18,009	16,179
Rhode Island	1,348	1,213	1,017	1,086	1,258	1,482	1,584	1,678	1,951	1,893
South Carolina	2,536	2,424	2,664	2,931	3,658	3,383	4,026	3,891	3,764	3,595
South Dakota	1,067	1,104	1,057	1,125	1,071	1,653	1,255	1,255	1,112	1,092
Tennessee	4,856	4,797	4,726	4,981	6,566	6,836	6,167	6,830	6,724	6,240
Texas	8,950	9,313	10,082	11,394	12,366	14,004	14,360	15,087	14,089	13,496
Utah	910	794	779	1,003	1,066	1,093	1,250	1,299	1,192	1,109
Vermont	432	414	414	453	515	603	672	681	649	535
Virginia	3,983	4,045	4,139	4,577	5,186	5,810	6,414	6,178	6,260	6,236
Washington	2,836	2,633	2,828	2,945	3,044	3,211	3,246	3,288	3,146	3,111
West Virginia	1,987	1,838	1,778	1,952	2,095	2,338	2,524	2,671	2,638	2,279
Wisconsin	5,573	4,275	4,406	4,650	5,630	5,962	6,330	7,475	6,924	6,163
Wyoming	337	442	484	478	562	705	594	550	479	481
American Samoa	14	16	16	16	16	13	16	11	11	15
Guam	60	60	0	19	20	69	69	68	113	102
Puerto Rico	3,642	3,561	2,918	2,980	3,408	3,120	3,575	4,157	3,754	4,354
Virgin Islands	56	73	50	47	55	55	75	77	111	111

[1] National and regional totals exclude American Samoa, Guam, Puerto Rico, and the Virgin Islands.

Table 20
TOTAL ENROLLMENTS IN BASIC BACCALAUREATE NURSING PROGRAMS,
BY NLN REGION AND STATE: 1986 TO 1995[1]

NLN REGION AND STATE	NUMBER OF TOTAL ENROLLMENTS[2]									
	1986	1987	1988	1989	1990	1991	1992	1993	1994	1995
United States	**81,602**	**73,621**	**70,078**	**74,865**	**81,788**	**90,877**	**102,128**	**110,693**	**112,659**	**109,505**
North Atlantic	23,065	19,710	17,695	17,742	18,563	20,450	24,777	27,797	28,628	27,686
Midwest	24,620	21,823	21,183	21,916	24,164	27,762	29,691	32,253	33,649	32,714
South	23,998	22,564	22,134	25,846	28,978	31,823	36,418	39,622	38,817	37,018
West	9,919	9,524	9,066	9,361	10,083	10,842	11,242	11,021	11,565	12,087
Alabama	2,276	1,991	1,904	2,040	2,160	2,723	3,546	4,040	4,070	3,734
Alaska	329	203	203	199	182	151	156	156	212	220
Arizona	765	591	595	546	523	548	644	801	843	877
Arkansas	594	580	549	672	740	856	969	1,091	1,229	884
California	4,258	4,309	3,947	3,990	4,173	4,654	4,747	4,676	4,855	4,962
Colorado	725	711	585	756	871	963	1,111	1,108	981	1,112
Connecticut	1,281	1,076	1,012	988	1,136	1,114	1,260	1,420	1,463	1,534
Delaware	625	467	411	419	460	343	633	759	819	719
District of Columbia	843	675	647	552	564	669	801	886	955	1,045
Florida	1,540	1,430	1,418	1,494	1,567	1,809	2,020	1,873	2,328	2,436
Georgia	1,025	901	988	1,215	1,372	1,589	1,810	2,136	2,249	2,261
Hawaii	228	401	354	284	162	220	288	429	548	696
Idaho	32	107	183	223	369	189	187	209	215	217
Illinois	3,826	3,249	3,059	3,028	3,131	3,667	4,201	4,787	5,977	6,020
Indiana	3,586	3,351	3,418	3,321	4,155	4,711	3,344	3,441	3,614	3,685
Iowa	1,057	821	779	788	859	1,006	1,182	1,308	1,338	1,320
Kansas	863	780	836	940	1,137	1,230	1,520	1,549	1,613	1,472
Kentucky	1,652	1,477	1,571	1,846	1,721	2,191	2,304	1,934	2,013	1,985
Louisiana	3,397	3,361	3,623	5,127	5,595	5,214	7,465	8,530	7,280	6,596
Maine	523	700	666	797	912	1,018	1,157	1,313	1,305	1,024
Maryland	1,166	968	758	819	770	974	1,244	1,385	1,543	1,525
Massachusetts	3,394	2,970	2,578	2,821	2,770	3,030	3,599	3,887	4,000	4,003
Michigan	3,283	3,157	3,096	2,867	2,991	3,341	3,717	3,582	3,699	3,816
Minnesota	1,138	1,046	844	895	903	1,072	1,140	1,307	1,159	1,178
Mississippi	1,179	998	958	995	1,311	1,428	1,494	1,399	1,170	1,063
Missouri	1,366	1,217	1,057	1,035	1,329	1,778	2,610	2,850	2,527	2,897
Montana	659	565	606	621	672	648	749	741	622	670
Nebraska	748	824	1,026	1,295	1,514	1,808	1,914	1,929	1,872	1,698
Nevada	181	193	231	281	338	376	255	267	271	266
New Hampshire	432	363	329	352	389	482	523	567	582	530
New Jersey	1,792	1,480	1,056	1,251	1,313	1,424	1,590	1,662	1,672	1,588
New Mexico	211	190	181	174	208	318	377	329	352	431
New York	6,826	5,793	4,981	4,603	4,389	5,000	6,469	7,701	8,158	8,154
North Carolina	1,623	1,563	1,348	1,409	1,776	1,745	2,081	2,265	2,239	2,287
North Dakota	606	537	551	738	862	722	913	808	777	732
Ohio	3,997	3,781	3,571	3,789	3,950	4,210	5,137	5,696	6,313	5,723
Oklahoma	740	933	780	947	1,076	1,271	1,357	1,266	1,233	1,242
Oregon	744	665	616	666	745	905	922	412	773	726
Pennsylvania	6,344	5,288	5,364	5,330	5,812	6,327	7,528	8,286	8,405	7,878
Rhode Island	754	682	470	461	616	809	966	1,060	1,019	946
South Carolina	1,195	994	997	1,049	1,139	1,337	1,777	1,753	1,774	1,618
South Dakota	624	594	555	632	606	1,165	744	592	554	609
Tennessee	1,785	1,667	1,629	1,662	2,547	2,418	1,868	2,544	2,761	2,806
Texas	3,792	3,747	3,676	4,238	4,492	5,350	5,224	5,890	5,371	5,256
Utah	407	395	378	415	523	442	515	544	576	577
Vermont	251	216	181	168	202	234	251	256	250	265
Virginia	1,488	1,339	1,327	1,611	1,850	1,911	2,165	2,255	2,255	2,235
Washington	1,179	977	962	971	1,079	1,179	1,166	1,227	1,194	1,218
West Virginia	546	615	608	722	862	1,007	1,094	1,261	1,302	1,090
Wisconsin	3,526	2,466	2,391	2,588	2,727	3,052	3,269	4,404	4,206	3,564
Wyoming	201	217	225	235	238	249	125	122	123	115
American Samoa	0	0	0	0	0	0	0	0	0	0
Guam	0	0	0	19	20	69	69	68	113	102
Puerto Rico	2,708	2,615	2,118	1,873	1,952	1,672	1,937	2,213	2,236	2,403
Virgin Islands	26	46	27	26	38	41	54	41	80	71

[1]National and regional totals exclude American Samoa, Guam, Puerto Rico, and the Virgin Islands.
[2]Includes basic students only.

Table 21
TOTAL ENROLLMENTS IN ASSOCIATE DEGREE NURSING PROGRAMS, BY NLN REGION AND STATE: 1986 TO 1995[1]

NLN REGION AND STATE	NUMBER OF TOTAL ENROLLMENTS									
	1986	1987	1988	1989	1990	1991	1992	1993	1994	1995
United States	**89,469**	**90,399**	**95,986**	**106,175**	**117,413**	**123,816**	**132,603**	**137,300**	**135,895**	**135,235**
North Atlantic	23,213	22,296	23,044	25,932	27,695	28,983	32,747	34,038	35,660	39,190
Midwest	22,013	22,497	23,215	26,084	29,737	30,330	31,590	32,876	32,385	31,644
South	30,104	31,166	34,576	38,281	43,550	47,296	50,835	52,583	50,773	48,304
West	14,139	14,440	15,151	15,878	16,431	17,207	17,431	17,803	17,077	16,097
Alabama	1,900	1,742	2,039	2,363	2,648	2,881	3,319	3,885	4,281	3,903
Alaska	63	65	66	75	86	80	72	68	57	55
Arizona	1,051	1,236	1,224	1,219	1,276	1,333	1,451	1,549	1,466	1,486
Arkansas	1,012	927	997	1,225	1,486	1,591	1,542	1,499	1,381	1,353
California	7,344	7,461	7,416	7,656	7,832	8,388	8,390	8,468	8,338	7,867
Colorado	709	682	751	836	835	860	826	988	922	871
Connecticut	742	680	703	761	638	1,038	1,113	970	976	966
Delaware	285	320	343	417	427	408	449	493	440	437
District of Columbia	212	79	152	152	146	90	76	97	96	96
Florida	3,854	3,905	4,299	4,672	5,383	5,799	5,966	6,446	6,399	6,247
Georgia	1,971	2,045	2,323	2,584	3,010	3,419	3,975	4,123	3,829	3,373
Hawaii	236	119	471	375	462	246	377	395	363	296
Idaho	438	443	442	487	516	533	497	483	489	453
Illinois	4,243	4,020	4,349	4,835	5,359	5,524	5,806	5,955	5,479	5,773
Indiana	1,954	1,969	2,339	2,695	3,604	3,125	3,297	3,363	3,493	3,709
Iowa	1,360	1,685	1,603	1,808	1,910	1,929	2,161	2,323	2,294	2,027
Kansas	822	947	1,063	1,269	1,512	1,446	1,465	1,576	1,459	1,398
Kentucky	1,869	2,073	2,230	2,404	2,794	3,336	3,610	3,729	3,581	3,192
Louisiana	973	993	1,260	1,510	1,676	2,168	2,797	3,633	2,769	2,536
Maine	329	284	318	356	438	490	670	656	629	604
Maryland	1,669	1,574	1,608	1,714	1,953	2,104	2,473	2,272	2,246	2,135
Massachusetts	2,586	2,328	2,274	2,560	2,718	2,876	3,068	3,202	3,148	3,058
Michigan	3,753	4,020	3,495	4,009	4,217	4,504	4,679	4,729	4,866	4,755
Minnesota	1,457	1,502	1,636	1,879	2,115	2,221	2,178	2,214	2,198	2,050
Mississippi	1,490	1,586	1,762	1,985	2,177	2,230	2,480	2,596	2,591	2,560
Missouri	1,617	1,567	1,561	1,664	1,857	2,032	2,260	2,479	2,689	2,542
Montana	228	174	262	275	244	240	245	233	293	215
Nebraska	112	156	97	232	414	478	520	498	483	458
Nevada	296	295	208	171	230	262	235	289	242	268
New Hampshire	328	401	467	553	727	761	885	855	836	839
New Jersey	2,069	2,048	2,280	2,311	2,455	2,707	2,932	2,946	2,909	2,709
New Mexico	546	730	806	898	1,012	1,019	1,009	1,018	1,076	879
New York	13,021	12,339	12,151	13,710	14,555	15,132	17,154	18,417	20,263	24,784
North Carolina	2,648	2,789	3,362	3,877	4,238	4,313	4,262	4,311	4,337	4,382
North Dakota	126	85	0	0	0	0	0	0	0	0
Ohio	4,453	4,478	4,826	5,332	5,580	5,900	5,933	6,311	6,283	5,967
Oklahoma	1,237	1,391	1,463	1,615	1,764	1,970	2,006	2,079	2,018	1,888
Oregon	932	955	979	1,081	1,106	1,107	1,045	1,068	907	916
Pennsylvania	3,007	3,202	3,659	4,280	4,722	4,536	5,463	5,468	5,146	4,584
Rhode Island	453	417	464	547	556	576	516	509	818	843
South Carolina	1,313	1,421	1,667	1,882	2,519	2,046	2,249	2,138	1,990	1,977
South Dakota	348	414	383	445	444	488	511	663	558	483
Tennessee	2,170	2,302	2,381	2,476	3,046	3,292	3,118	3,102	2,920	2,714
Texas	4,951	5,340	6,142	6,830	7,482	8,225	8,698	8,760	8,297	7,857
Utah	503	399	401	588	543	651	735	755	616	532
Vermont	181	198	233	285	313	369	421	425	399	270
Virginia	1,813	2,015	2,038	2,075	2,299	2,743	3,061	2,755	2,935	3,058
Washington	1,657	1,656	1,866	1974	1,965	2,032	2,080	2,061	1,952	1,893
West Virginia	1,234	1,063	1,005	1,069	1,075	1,179	1,279	1,255	1,199	1,129
Wisconsin	1,768	1,654	1,863	1,916	2,725	2,683	2,780	2,765	2,583	2,482
Wyoming	136	225	259	243	324	456	469	428	356	366
American Samoa	14	16	16	16	16	13	16	11	11	15
Guam	60	60	0	0	0	0	0	0	0	0
Puerto Rico	934	946	800	1,107	1,456	1,448	1,638	1,944	1,518	1,951
Virgin Islands	30	27	23	21	17	14	21	36	31	40

[1] National and regional totals exclude American Samoa, Guam, Puerto Rico, and the Virgin Islands.

Table 22

TOTAL ENROLLMENTS IN DIPLOMA NURSING PROGRAMS, BY NLN REGION AND STATE: 1986 TO 1995[1]

NLN REGION AND STATE	NUMBER OF TOTAL ENROLLMENTS									
	1986	1987	1988	1989	1990	1991	1992	1993	1994	1995
United States	**22,641**	**18,927**	**18,860**	**20,418**	**21,969**	**22,905**	**23,252**	**22,235**	**19,796**	**16,479**
North Atlantic	10,067	8,515	8,794	9,641	10,415	10,843	10,988	10,436	9,800	8,468
Midwest	7,958	6,130	5,559	5,665	5,781	6,008	6,259	6,092	4,970	4,106
South	4,214	3,944	4,202	4,755	5,323	5,585	5,543	5,325	4,694	3,660
West	402	338	305	357	450	469	462	382	332	245
Alabama	124	66	60	59	78	100	97	83	29	0
Alaska	0	0	0	0	0	0	0	0	0	0
Arizona	0	0	0	0	0	0	0	0	0	0
Arkansas	330	422	624	730	1,042	1,181	1,223	944	737	643
California	390	338	305	357	450	469	462	382	332	245
Colorado	12	0	0	0	0	0	0	0	0	0
Connecticut	528	511	553	622	732	632	361	370	357	277
Delaware	47	42	46	43	50	58	73	75	73	72
District of Columbia	0	0	0	0	0	0	0	0	0	0
Florida	151	140	160	205	231	192	180	191	191	126
Georgia	282	239	221	143	68	18	0	0	0	0
Hawaii	0	0	0	0	0	0	0	0	0	0
Idaho	0	0	0	0	0	0	0	0	0	0
Illinois	1,177	818	706	669	681	628	745	780	648	595
Indiana	720	510	250	203	157	191	230	289	263	200
Iowa	549	411	435	530	651	770	937	888	717	657
Kansas	90	64	52	63	72	49	30	0	0	0
Kentucky	0	0	0	0	0	0	0	0	0	0
Louisiana	711	603	579	526	349	222	74	77	81	80
Maine	58	17	0	0	0	0	0	0	0	0
Maryland	262	233	263	305	332	346	354	358	310	239
Massachusetts	1,139	941	741	851	1,025	1,156	1,216	1,224	1,186	1,086
Michigan	504	376	337	343	367	425	469	485	412	159
Minnesota	64	0	0	0	0	0	0	0	0	0
Mississippi	0	0	0	0	0	0	0	0	0	0
Missouri	1,235	1,091	1,084	1,244	1,235	1,222	1,086	1,008	801	579
Montana	0	0	0	0	0	0	0	0	0	0
Nebraska	406	189	73	76	83	83	101	125	103	117
Nevada	0	0	0	0	0	0	0	0	0	0
New Hampshire	59	39	9	0	0	0	0	0	0	0
New Jersey	2,081	1,882	2,306	2,397	2,650	3,009	3,266	3,278	3,117	2,782
New Mexico	0	0	0	0	0	0	0	0	0	0
New York	1,533	1,134	973	1,101	1,112	978	892	538	495	430
North Carolina	329	327	376	566	663	663	657	728	675	466
North Dakota	133	28	0	0	0	0	0	0	0	0
Ohio	2,706	2,392	2,351	2,343	2,336	2,413	2,380	2,211	1,891	1,682
Oklahoma	0	0	0	0	0	0	0	0	0	0
Oregon	0	0	0	0	0	0	0	0	0	0
Pennsylvania	4,481	3,835	4,083	4,549	4,760	4,913	5,078	4,842	4,458	3,717
Rhode Island	141	114	83	78	86	97	102	109	114	104
South Carolina	28	9	0	0	0	0	0	0	0	0
South Dakota	95	96	119	48	21	0	0	0	0	0
Tennessee	901	828	716	843	973	1,126	1,181	1,184	1,043	720
Texas	207	226	264	326	392	429	438	437	421	383
Utah	0	0	0	0	0	0	0	0	0	0
Vermont	0	0	0	0	0	0	0	0	0	0
Virginia	682	691	774	891	1,037	1,156	1,188	1,168	1,070	943
Washington	0	0	0	0	0	0	0	0	0	0
West Virginia	207	160	165	161	158	152	151	155	137	60
Wisconsin	279	155	152	146	178	227	281	306	135	117
Wyoming	0	0	0	0	0	0	0	0	0	0
American Samoa	0	0	0	0	0	0	0	0	0	0
Guam	0	0	0	0	0	0	0	0	0	0
Puerto Rico	0	0	0	0	0	0	0	0	0	0
Virgin Islands	0	0	0	0	0	0	0	0	0	0

[1] National and regional totals exclude American Samoa, Guam, Puerto Rico, and the Virgin Islands.

Table 23
BASIC AND RN STUDENT ENROLLMENTS IN BACCALAUREATE NURSING PROGRAMS: 1986 TO 1995[1]

YEAR	ENROLLMENTS IN BACCALAUREATE NURSING PROGRAMS			
	Total Enrollments	Basic Programs		BRN* Programs
		Basic Students	RN Students	RN Students
1986	127,957	81,602	25,247	21,108
1987	119,996	73,621	26,503	19,872
1988	113,105	70,078	25,597	17,430
1989	116,539	74,865	24,524	17,150
1990	122,504	81,788	23,777	16,939
1991	130,195	90,877	22,634	16,684
1992	142,494	102,128	22,399	17,967
1993	151,566	110,693	23,075	17,798
1994	155,655	112,659	25,536	17,460
1995	156,605	109,505	26,057	21,043

[1] Excludes American Samoa, Guam, Puerto Rico, and the Virgin Islands.
* BRN programs are baccalaureate programs that admit only RNs.

Table 24
FULL-TIME AND PART-TIME ENROLLMENTS OF BASIC AND RN STUDENTS IN BACCALAUREATE NURSING PROGRAMS: 1991 TO 1995[1]

YEAR AND TYPE OF STUDENT	ENROLLMENTS IN BACCALAUREATE NURSING PROGRAMS		
	Total	Full Time	Part Time
1991 (Total)	**130,195**	**86,094**	**44,101**
Basic Students	90,877	77,152	13,725
RNs in Basic Programs	22,634	6,016	16,618
RNs in BRN* Programs	16,684	2,926	13,758
1992 (Total)	**142,494**	**95,745**	**46,749**
Basic Students	102,128	88,002	14,126
RNs in Basic Programs	22,399	4,353	18,046
RNs in BRN* Programs	17,967	3,390	14,577
1993 (Total)	**151,566**	**104,793**	**46,773**
Basic Students	110,693	96,316	14,377
RNs in Basic Programs	23,075	4,617	18,458
RNs in BRN* Programs	17,798	3,860	13,938
1994 (Total)	**155,655**	**105,021**	**50,634**
Basic Students	112,659	96,653	16,006
RNs in Basic Programs	25,536	4,549	20,987
RNs in BRN* Programs	17,460	3,819	13,641
1995 (Total)	**156,605**	**104,413**	**52,192**
Basic Students	109,505	94,797	14,708
RNs in Basic Programs	26,057	4,649	21,408
RNs in BRN* Programs	21,043	4,967	16,076

[1] Excludes American Samoa, Guam, Puerto Rico, and the Virgin Islands.
*BRN programs are baccalaureate programs that admit only RNs.

Table 25
TOTAL ENROLLMENTS IN BACCALAUREATE NURSING PROGRAMS, BY NLN REGION AND STATE:
1991 TO 1995[1]

NLN REGION AND STATE	ENROLLMENTS IN BACCALAUREATE NURSING PROGRAMS [2]									
	1991		1992		1993		1994		1995	
	Total	RNs Only	Total	RNs Only	Total	RNs Only	Total	RNs Only	Total	RNs Only
United States	**130,195**	**39,318**	**142,494**	**40,366**	**151,566**	**40,873**	**155,655**	**42,996**	**156,605**	**47,100**
North Atlantic	34,768	14,318	39,973	15,196	43,267	15,470	46,490	17,862	46,399	18,713
Midwest	38,916	11,154	40,577	10,886	43,225	10,972	45,071	11,422	44,317	11,603
South	39,761	7,938	44,153	7,735	47,651	8,029	47,656	8,839	46,989	9,971
West	16,750	5,908	17,791	6,549	17,423	6,402	16,438	4,873	18,900	6,813
Alabama	3,173	450	3,969	423	4,424	384	4,501	431	4,269	535
Alaska	165	14	167	11	165	9	222	10	227	7
Arizona	1,493	945	1,767	1,123	2,062	1,261	2,350	1,507	2,718	1,841
Arkansas	930	74	1,072	103	1,188	97	1,366	137	973	89
California	8,015	3,361	8,197	3,450	7,988	3,312	5,990	1,135	7,815	2,853
Colorado	1,314	351	1,602	491	1,642	534	1,594	613	1,714	602
Connecticut	1,851	737	1,963	703	2,182	762	2,415	952	2,466	932
Delaware	618	275	996	363	1,289	530	1,545	726	1,513	794
District of Columbia	769	100	916	115	968	82	1,032	77	1,106	61
Florida	3,114	1,305	3,247	1,227	3,229	1,356	3,868	1,540	3,960	1,524
Georgia	2,055	466	2,313	503	2,702	566	2,879	630	2,962	701
Hawaii	398	178	422	134	562	133	673	1257	786	90
Idaho	272	83	310	123	339	130	339	124	258	41
Illinois	5,030	1,363	5,703	1,502	6,176	1,389	7,466	1,489	7,569	1,549
Indiana	5,748	1,037	4,360	1,016	4,427	986	4,694	1,080	5,047	1,362
Iowa	1,624	618	2,043	861	2,311	1,003	1,876	538	1,845	525
Kansas	1,733	503	2,151	631	2,148	599	2,234	621	1,758	286
Kentucky	2,872	681	2,825	521	2,494	560	2,456	443	2,523	538
Louisiana	5,531	317	7,803	338	8,867	337	7,694	414	7,060	464
Maine	1,241	223	1,575	418	1,825	512	1,872	567	1,681	657
Maryland	1,527	553	1,939	695	1,995	610	2,170	627	2,354	829
Massachusetts	4,808	1,778	5,261	1,662	5,177	1,290	5,820	1,820	5,836	1,833
Michigan	5,206	1,865	5,354	1,637	5,187	1,605	5,101	1,402	5,347	1,531
Minnesota	1,701	629	1,706	566	1,875	568	1,775	616	1,791	613
Mississippi	1,511	83	1,573	79	1,515	116	1,368	198	1,260	197
Missouri	3,141	1,363	3,941	1,331	4,148	1,298	4,470	1,943	4,874	1,977
Montana	686	38	783	34	770	29	727	105	766	96
Nebraska	2,415	607	2,376	462	2,430	501	2,256	384	2,197	499
Nevada	440	64	302	47	311	44	308	37	305	39
New Hampshire	756	274	744	221	826	259	1,212	630	1,110	580
New Jersey	2,772	1,348	2,932	1,342	3,020	1,358	3,301	1,629	3,444	1,856
New Mexico	571	253	639	262	593	264	626	274	797	366
New York	10,979	5,979	12,938	6,469	14,378	6,677	14,916	6,758	15,618	7,464
North Carolina	2,362	617	2,793	712	3,005	740	3,059	820	3,256	969
North Dakota	822	100	974	61	859	51	877	100	839	107
Ohio	6,114	1,904	7,011	1,874	7,486	1,790	8,376	2,063	7,739	2,016
Oklahoma	1,455	184	1,501	144	1,403	137	1,393	160	1,405	163
Oregon	986	81	1,123	201	431	19	958	185	893	167
Pennsylvania	9,610	3,283	11,089	3,561	11,968	3,682	12,808	4,403	12,154	4,276
Rhode Island	956	147	1,122	156	1,169	109	1,152	133	997	51
South Carolina	1,640	303	2,026	249	2,053	300	2,064	290	1,976	358
South Dakota	1,418	253	872	128	825	233	673	119	710	101
Tennessee	3,122	704	2,472	604	3,171	627	3,481	720	3,439	633
Texas	6,287	937	6,156	932	6,939	1,049	6,365	994	6,162	906
Utah	612	170	732	217	803	259	833	257	809	232
Vermont	408	174	437	186	465	209	417	167	474	209
Virginia	2,735	824	2,896	731	2,993	738	3,212	957	3,862	1,627
Washington	1,524	345	1,615	449	1,627	400	1,683	489	1,666	448
West Virginia	1,447	440	1,568	474	1,673	412	1,780	478	1,528	438
Wisconsin	3,964	912	4,086	817	5,353	949	5,273	1,067	4,601	1,037
Wyoming	274	25	132	7	130	8	135	12	146	31
American Samoa	0	0	0	0	0	0	0	0	0	0
Guam	108	39	69	0	79	11	123	10	107	5
Puerto Rico	1,966	294	2,253	316	2,471	258	2,517	281	2,685	282
Virgin Islands	52	11	60	6	45	4	91	11	73	2

[1] National and regional totals exclude American Samoa, Guam, Puerto Rico, and the Virgin Islands.
[2] Totals include RNs in basic programs, RNs in BRN programs, and basic BSN students.

Table 26
GRADUATIONS FROM BASIC RN PROGRAMS AND PERCENTAGE CHANGE FROM PREVIOUS YEAR, BY TYPE OF PROGRAM: 1975-76 TO 1994-95[1]

ACADEMIC YEAR	ALL BASIC RN PROGRAMS		BACCALAUREATE PROGRAMS		ASSOCIATE DEGREE PROGRAMS		DIPLOMA PROGRAMS	
	Number of Graduations	Percent Change	Number of Graduations	Percent Change	Number of Graduations	Percent Change	Number of Graduations	Percent Change
1975-76	77,065	+4.3	22,579	+11.9	34,625	+7.6	19,861	-7.9
1976-77	77,755	+0.9	23,452	+3.9	36,289	+4.8	18,014	-9.3
1977-78	77,874	+0.1	24,187	+3.1	36,556	+0.7	17,131	-4.9
1978-79	77,132	-1.0	25,048	+3.6	36,264	-0.8	15,820	-7.7
1979-80	75,523	-2.1	24,994	-0.2	36,034	-0.6	14,495	-8.4
1980-81	73,985	-2.0	24,370	-2.5	36,712	+1.9	12,903	-11.0
1981-82	74,052	+0.1	24,081	-1.2	38,289	+4.3	11,682	-9.5
1982-83	77,408	+4.5	23,855	-0.9	41,849	+9.3	11,704	+0.2
1983-84	80,312	+3.8	23,718	-0.6	44,394	+6.1	12,200	+4.2
1984-85	82,075	+2.2	24,975	+5.3	45,208	+1.8	11,892	-2.5
1985-86	77,027	-6.2	25,170	+0.8	41,333	-8.6	10,524	-11.5
1986-87	70,561	-8.4	23,761	-5.6	38,528	-6.8	8,272	-21.4
1987-88	64,839	-8.0	21,504	-9.5	37,397	-2.9	5,938	-28.2
1988-89	61,660	-4.9	18,997	-11.6	37,837	+1.2	4,826	-18.7
1989-90	66,088	+7.2	18,571	-2.2	42,318	+11.8	5,199	+7.7
1990-91	72,230	+9.3	19,264	+3.7	46,794	+10.6	6,172	+18.7
1991-92	80,839	+11.9	21,415	+11.2	52,896	+13.0	6,528	+5.8
1992-93	88,149	+9.0	24,442	+14.1	56,770	+7.3	6,937	+6.3
1993-94	94,870	+7.6	28,912	+18.3	58,839	+3.6	7,119	+2.6
1994-95	97,052	+2.3	31,254	+8.1	58,749	-0.1	7,049	-1.0

[1] Excludes American Samoa, Guam, Puerto Rico, and the Virgin Islands.

Table 27
GRADUATIONS FROM PUBLIC AND PRIVATE BASIC RN PROGRAMS, BY TYPE OF PROGRAM: 1985-86 TO 1994-95[1]

PUBLIC AND PRIVATE NURSING PROGRAMS	NUMBER OF GRADUATIONS									
	1985-86	1986-87	1987-88	1988-89	1989-90	1990-91	1991-92	1992-93	1993-94	1994-95
All Programs	**77,027**	**70,561**	**64,839**	**61,660**	**66,088**	**72,230**	**80,839**	**88,149**	**94,870**	**97,052**
Public	54,456	50,865	48,608	47,644	51,926	57,892	64,405	70,152	73,610	71,841
Private	22,571	19,696	16,231	14,016	14,162	14,338	16,434	17,997	21,260	25,211
Baccalaureate	25,170	23,761	21,504	18,997	18,571	19,264	21,415	24,442	28,912	31,254
Public	15,977	14,746	13,568	12,203	12,434	13,073	14,498	16,588	18,902	19,427
Private	9,193	9,015	7,936	6,794	6,137	6,191	6,917	7,854	10,010	11,827
Associate Degree	41,333	38,528	37,397	37,837	42,318	46,794	52,896	56,770	58,839	58,749
Public	36,806	34,696	33,795	34,460	38,439	43,337	48,535	52,017	53,294	51,448
Private	4,527	3,832	3,602	3,377	3,879	3,457	4,361	4,753	5,545	7,301
Diploma	10,524	8,272	5,938	4,826	5,199	6,172	6,528	6,937	7,119	7,049
Public	1,673	1,423	1,245	981	1,053	1,482	1,372	1,547	1,414	966
Private	8,851	6,849	4,693	3,845	4,146	4,690	5,156	5,390	5,705	6,083

[1] Excludes American Samoa, Guam, Puerto Rico, and the Virgin Islands.

Table 28
GRADUATIONS FROM ALL BASIC RN PROGRAMS, BY NLN REGION AND STATE: 1985-86 TO 1994-95[1]

NLN REGION AND STATE	NUMBER OF GRADUATIONS									
	1985-86	1986-87	1987-88	1988-89	1989-90	1990-91	1991-92	1992-93	1993-94	1994-95
United States	**77,027**	**70,561**	**64,839**	**61,660**	**66,088**	**72,230**	**80,839**	**88,149**	**94,870**	**97,052**
North Atlantic	19,622	18,274	16,617	15,054	15,347	16,278	18,762	20,116	21,414	22,484
Midwest	23,378	20,664	18,072	17,264	18,354	19,961	21,900	24,137	25,713	26,865
South	23,250	21,397	20,123	19,768	21,982	25,214	28,622	32,047	35,133	35,552
West	10,777	10,226	10,027	9,574	10,405	10,777	11,555	11,849	12,610	12,151
Alabama	1,857	1,587	1,430	1,354	1,425	1,565	1,867	1,970	2,642	2,843
Alaska	61	51	46	64	62	51	77	78	79	74
Arizona	797	795	767	784	807	796	792	918	1,064	1,066
Arkansas	771	726	685	687	878	1,039	1,224	1,216	1,254	1,252
California	5,566	5,125	4,969	4,716	4,956	5,045	5,245	5,295	5,591	5,431
Colorado	585	521	552	524	584	751	845	912	966	877
Connecticut	917	814	733	663	710	737	878	811	823	896
Delaware	311	308	278	267	273	272	284	277	358	353
District of Columbia	332	279	246	231	191	169	188	181	234	246
Florida	2,995	2,655	2,715	2,504	2,677	3,064	3,496	3,834	4,025	4,285
Georgia	1,547	1,432	1,236	1,206	1,446	1,604	1,848	2,164	2,467	2,681
Hawaii	172	133	202	170	250	296	240	276	259	260
Idaho	249	212	228	214	270	291	336	318	325	312
Illinois	4,012	3,370	2,974	2,822	2,945	3,164	3,266	4,131	4,152	4,240
Indiana	2,230	2,026	1,755	1,734	1,747	1,881	2,034	2,236	2,537	3,232
Iowa	1,566	1,385	1,135	1,173	1,234	1,293	1,483	1,585	1,656	1,746
Kansas	1,051	915	843	812	1,171	1,214	1,191	1,312	1,359	1,403
Kentucky	1,287	1,092	1,148	1,193	1,253	1,424	1,674	1,994	2,190	2,086
Louisiana	1,000	998	999	994	980	1,216	1,201	1,700	1,811	1,847
Maine	379	364	288	310	269	326	400	483	594	633
Maryland	1,357	1,205	1,026	920	1,013	1,107	1,323	1,463	1,665	1,599
Massachusetts	2,420	2,386	2,029	1,685	1,726	1,865	2,016	2,272	2,536	2,604
Michigan	3,136	3,119	2,763	2,701	2,583	2,688	3,016	3,259	3,322	3,321
Minnesota	1,500	1,246	1,125	1,141	1,170	1,385	1,502	1,599	1,664	1,604
Mississippi	1,013	1,035	851	799	911	1,147	1,226	1,369	1,571	1,572
Missouri	1,859	1,461	1,397	1,358	1,456	1,771	1,963	2,175	2,479	2,565
Montana	258	245	203	208	225	207	243	215	267	285
Nebraska	503	430	288	321	347	430	613	703	844	927
Nevada	171	153	182	149	153	173	236	228	266	231
New Hampshire	334	311	305	275	313	331	359	503	485	498
New Jersey	2,072	1,863	1,678	1,570	1,640	1,766	2,027	2,258	2,372	2,319
New Mexico	407	430	385	418	550	499	534	566	601	582
New York	6,812	6,467	6,052	5,712	5,582	5,905	6,867	7,116	7,402	8,232
North Carolina	1,967	1,759	1,722	1,760	2,005	2,342	2,547	2,910	3,063	3,100
North Dakota	419	310	179	202	186	215	271	288	294	300
Ohio	4,782	4,355	3,753	3,459	3,726	3,898	4,350	4,566	4,874	4,964
Oklahoma	782	805	786	902	881	1,088	1,181	1,282	1,413	1,349
Oregon	740	748	755	643	697	670	776	838	782	795
Pennsylvania	5,304	4,844	4,459	3,835	4,139	4,315	5,141	5,568	5,763	5,936
Rhode Island	532	457	404	393	364	439	430	421	625	624
South Carolina	889	884	846	863	886	1,056	1,096	1,217	1,257	1,254
South Dakota	421	324	378	322	365	442	441	414	463	425
Tennessee	1,850	1,673	1,431	1,296	1,436	1,571	1,936	2,252	2,411	2,632
Texas	3,425	3,347	3,186	3,320	3,951	4,605	5,314	5,720	6,049	5,875
Utah	373	402	454	477	475	600	664	644	730	727
Vermont	209	181	145	113	140	153	172	226	222	143
Virginia	1,677	1,465	1,459	1,356	1,516	1,618	1,913	2,082	2,374	2,314
Washington	1,263	1,293	1,149	1,056	1,185	1,195	1,309	1,287	1,429	1,299
West Virginia	833	734	603	614	724	768	776	874	941	863
Wisconsin	1,899	1,723	1,482	1,219	1,424	1,580	1,770	1,869	2,069	2,138
Wyoming	135	118	135	151	191	203	258	274	251	212
American Samoa	10	10	10	10	12	13	12	6	6	7
Guam	12	12	0	0	20	0	0	7	16	11
Puerto Rico	1,017	1,045	908	962	1,022	989	914	951	915	1,196
Virgin Islands	13	12	17	11	6	12	14	10	14	15

[1] National and regional totals exclude American Samoa, Guam, Puerto Rico, and the Virgin Islands.

Table 29
GRADUATIONS FROM BASIC BACCALAUREATE NURSING PROGRAMS,
BY NLN REGION AND STATE: 1985-86 TO 1994-95[1]

NLN REGION AND STATE	NUMBER OF GRADUATIONS[2]									
	1985-86	1986-87	1987-88	1988-89	1989-90	1990-91	1991-92	1992-93	1993-94	1994-95
United States	**25,170**	**23,761**	**21,504**	**18,997**	**18,571**	**19,264**	**21,415**	**24,442**	**28,912**	**31,254**
North Atlantic	6,744	6,320	5,720	4,802	4,208	4,001	4,294	4,959	5,793	6,556
Midwest	7,600	7,218	6,430	5,756	5,670	5,861	6,523	7,364	8,856	9,746
South	7,562	6,970	6,423	5,804	5,868	6,521	7,570	8,794	10,433	11,033
West	3,264	3,253	2,931	2,635	2,825	2,881	3,028	3,325	3,830	3,919
Alabama	781	688	568	511	491	481	522	553	912	1,003
Alaska	38	26	26	34	32	21	32	48	46	47
Arizona	251	279	247	230	240	201	186	241	269	317
Arkansas	207	188	200	152	196	185	241	256	297	332
California	1,362	1,394	1,283	1,163	1,242	1,221	1,184	1,285	1,500	1,515
Colorado	266	179	210	179	235	297	364	414	461	419
Connecticut	363	302	286	260	233	214	287	278	292	382
Delaware	166	167	137	105	93	67	90	85	121	161
District of Columbia	294	218	191	176	146	125	170	155	200	212
Florida	570	561	521	503	513	500	619	724	695	799
Georgia	425	446	415	326	397	453	483	582	777	841
Hawaii	65	89	90	40	72	134	66	96	98	121
Idaho	31	34	26	32	56	71	80	74	73	84
Illinois	1,185	1,156	984	943	929	841	892	1,019	1,345	1,444
Indiana	899	784	774	701	641	632	722	796	975	1,380
Iowa	438	410	322	254	231	239	271	304	324	396
Kansas	447	408	291	281	345	386	395	536	590	637
Kentucky	498	319	365	342	331	308	359	464	553	501
Louisiana	438	450	490	505	472	608	601	818	872	937
Maine	171	176	166	159	107	140	165	198	252	270
Maryland	393	379	345	282	262	278	356	390	532	559
Massachusetts	917	862	796	631	598	531	591	684	811	755
Michigan	902	897	850	862	728	753	801	969	933	1,009
Minnesota	507	466	415	322	339	389	427	540	578	522
Mississippi	356	359	309	208	250	322	395	425	507	556
Missouri	432	319	352	333	323	333	459	575	710	850
Montana	175	174	144	139	137	100	140	109	152	165
Nebraska	160	152	185	192	227	259	367	391	548	642
Nevada	43	33	35	34	45	61	89	99	98	111
New Hampshire	124	118	97	86	76	81	77	119	120	124
New Jersey	419	413	382	347	318	294	265	339	391	361
New Mexico	86	73	71	50	58	46	59	69	93	93
New York	1,982	1,959	1,724	1,468	1,227	1,092	1,131	1,305	1,628	1,936
North Carolina	626	558	508	440	369	450	586	702	724	779
North Dakota	192	198	179	202	186	215	271	288	294	300
Ohio	1,315	1,326	1,198	1,006	1,008	1,003	1,012	1,116	1,477	1,458
Oklahoma	339	314	254	327	270	316	338	416	439	411
Oregon	266	288	248	221	216	221	270	284	282	314
Pennsylvania	1,957	1,813	1,677	1,370	1,257	1,289	1,358	1,556	1,697	2,082
Rhode Island	279	214	193	154	121	120	123	184	231	224
South Carolina	363	354	309	279	268	277	247	328	375	430
South Dakota	175	157	152	112	121	185	224	117	199	186
Tennessee	537	449	415	336	433	405	552	690	844	1,030
Texas	1,293	1,232	1,105	1,050	1,076	1,268	1,504	1,697	1,966	1,957
Utah	168	192	162	146	146	170	175	188	236	242
Vermon	72	78	71	46	32	48	37	56	50	49
Virginia	573	528	476	426	406	464	541	533	635	588
Washington	461	453	366	333	299	305	332	363	467	439
West Virginia	163	145	143	117	134	206	226	216	305	310
Wisconsin	948	945	728	548	592	626	682	713	883	922
Wyoming	52	39	23	34	47	33	51	55	55	52
American Samoa	0	0	0	0	0	0	0	0	0	0
Guam	0	0	0	0	20	0	0	7	16	11
Puerto Rico	625	553	572	626	569	527	465	412	438	563
Virgin Islands	4	7	9	3	4	6	6	4	5	8

[1] National and regional totals exclude American Samoa, Guam, Puerto Rico, and the Virgin Islands.
[2] Includes basic students only.

Table 30
GRADUATIONS FROM ASSOCIATE DEGREE NURSING PROGRAMS,
BY NLN REGION AND STATE: 1985-86 TO 1994-95[1]

NLN REGION AND STATE	NUMBER OF GRADUATIONS									
	1985-86	1986-87	1987-88	1988-89	1989-90	1990-91	1991-92	1992-93	1993-94	1994-95
United States	**41,333**	**38,528**	**37,397**	**37,837**	**42,318**	**46,794**	**52,896**	**56,770**	**58,839**	**58,749**
North Atlantic	8,791	8,530	8,164	8,101	8,778	9,463	11,381	12,040	12,425	12,689
Midwest	11,512	10,418	9,734	10,050	11,234	12,343	13,656	14,767	14,884	15,243
South	13,744	12,794	12,570	12,884	14,851	17,264	19,524	21,656	22,926	22,748
West	7,286	6,786	6,929	6,802	7,455	7,724	8,335	8,307	8,604	8,069
Alabama	972	865	842	825	918	1,072	1,307	1,384	1,697	1,840
Alaska	23	25	20	30	30	30	45	30	33	27
Arizona	546	516	520	554	567	595	606	677	795	749
Arkansas	475	435	395	400	494	643	731	687	668	636
California	4,002	3,544	3,519	3,416	3,589	3,652	3,869	3,793	3,915	3,753
Colorado	294	342	342	345	349	454	481	498	505	458
Connecticut	310	309	282	227	281	300	405	380	376	346
Delaware	133	129	133	153	172	195	186	184	213	176
District of Columbia	38	61	55	55	45	44	18	26	34	34
Florida	2,315	2,017	2,143	1,944	2,098	2,457	2,790	3,037	3,243	3,391
Georgia	981	820	745	826	988	1,101	1,365	1,582	1,690	1,840
Hawaii	107	44	112	130	178	162	174	180	161	139
Idaho	218	178	202	182	214	220	256	244	252	228
Illinois	2,096	1,818	1,712	1,724	1,875	2,105	2,281	2,904	2,582	2,614
Indiana	1,078	984	845	952	1,034	1,199	1,289	1,405	1,507	1,767
Iowa	778	795	699	807	893	923	1,043	1,038	1,078	1,084
Kansas	511	470	519	521	809	808	772	776	769	766
Kentucky	789	773	783	851	922	1,116	1,315	1,530	1,637	1,585
Louisiana	344	326	328	295	341	452	574	847	902	875
Maine	161	163	122	151	162	186	235	285	342	363
Maryland	825	732	609	564	653	739	847	942	997	934
Massachusetts	995	1,129	942	890	904	1,048	1,100	1,222	1,346	1,413
Michigan	1,980	2,016	1,755	1,727	1,744	1,802	2,045	2,088	2,164	2,163
Minnesota	901	780	710	819	831	996	1,075	1,059	1,086	1,082
Mississippi	657	676	542	591	661	825	831	944	1,064	1,016
Missouri	804	677	666	686	775	943	1,100	1,111	1,347	1,325
Montana	83	71	59	69	88	107	103	106	115	120
Nebraska	65	56	41	72	80	131	193	255	235	197
Nevada	128	120	147	115	108	112	147	129	168	120
New Hampshire	187	179	179	189	237	250	282	384	365	374
New Jersey	975	820	794	783	904	947	1,139	1,211	1,220	1,200
New Mexico	321	357	314	368	492	453	475	497	508	489
New York	4,201	3,985	4,002	4,025	4,093	4,478	5,365	5,634	5,576	6,102
North Carolina	1,159	1,070	1,126	1,254	1,517	1,695	1,731	1,982	2,110	2,101
North Dakota	87	61	0	0	0	0	0	0	0	0
Ohio	2,199	1,926	1,868	1,896	2,163	2,281	2,585	2,720	2,706	2,838
Oklahoma	443	491	532	575	611	772	843	866	974	938
Oregon	474	460	507	422	481	449	506	554	500	481
Pennsylvania	1,466	1,450	1,412	1,347	1,655	1,607	2,231	2,338	2,417	2,214
Rhode Island	188	202	169	214	217	303	285	206	364	373
South Carolina	514	524	537	584	618	779	849	889	882	824
South Dakota	202	139	209	193	224	239	217	297	264	239
Tennessee	854	840	807	824	884	1,014	1,151	1,308	1,256	1,222
Texas	2,023	2,013	1,973	2,161	2,728	3,179	3,605	3,821	3,889	3,710
Utah	205	210	292	331	329	430	489	456	494	485
Vermont	137	103	74	67	108	105	135	170	172	94
Virginia	825	709	799	775	909	935	1,105	1,248	1,351	1,355
Washington	802	840	783	723	886	890	977	924	962	860
West Virginia	568	503	409	415	509	485	480	589	566	481
Wisconsin	811	696	710	653	806	916	1,056	1,114	1,146	1,168
Wyoming	83	79	112	117	144	170	207	219	196	160
American Samoa	10	10	10	10	12	13	12	6	6	7
Guam	12	12	0	0	0	0	0	0	0	0
Puerto Rico	392	492	336	336	453	462	449	539	477	633
Virgin Islands	9	5	8	8	2	6	8	6	9	7

[1] National and regional totals exclude American Samoa, Guam, Puerto Rico, and the Virgin Islands.

Table 31

GRAUATIONS FROM DIPLOMA NURSING PROGRAMS, BY NLN REGION AND STATE: 1985-86 TO 1994-95[1]

NLN REGION AND STATE	NUMBER OF GRADUATIONS									
	1985-86	1986-87	1987-88	1988-89	1989-90	1990-91	1991-92	1992-93	1993-94	1994-95
United States	**10,524**	**8,272**	**5,938**	**4,826**	**5,199**	**6,172**	**6,528**	**6,937**	**7,119**	**7,049**
North Atlantic	4,087	3,424	2,733	2,151	2,361	2,814	3,087	3,117	3,196	3,239
Midwest	4,266	3,028	1,908	1,458	1,450	1,757	1,721	2,006	1,973	1,876
South	1,944	1,633	1,130	1,080	1,263	1,429	1,528	1,597	1,774	1,771
West	277	187	167	137	125	172	192	217	176	163
Alabama	104	34	20	18	16	12	38	33	33	0
Alaska	0	0	0	0	0	0	0	0	0	0
Arizona	0	0	0	0	0	0	0	0	0	0
Arkansas	89	103	90	135	188	211	252	273	289	284
California	202	187	167	137	125	172	192	217	176	163
Colorado	25	0	0	0	0	0	0	0	0	0
Connecticut	244	203	165	176	196	223	186	153	155	168
Delaware	12	12	8	9	8	10	8	8	24	16
District of Columbia	0	0	0	0	0	0	0	0	0	0
Florida	110	77	51	57	66	107	87	73	87	95
Georgia	141	166	76	54	61	50	0	0	0	0
Hawaii	0	0	0	0	0	0	0	0	0	0
Idaho	0	0	0	0	0	0	0	0	0	0
Illinois	731	396	278	155	141	218	93	208	225	182
Indiana	253	258	136	81	72	50	23	35	55	85
Iowa	350	180	114	112	110	131	169	243	254	266
Kansas	93	37	33	10	17	20	24	0	0	0
Kentucky	0	0	0	0	0	0	0	0	0	0
Louisiana	218	222	181	194	167	156	26	35	37	35
Maine	47	25	0	0	0	0	0	0	0	0
Maryland	139	94	72	74	98	90	120	131	136	106
Massachusetts	508	395	291	164	224	286	325	366	379	436
Michigan	254	206	158	112	111	133	170	202	225	149
Minnesota	92	0	0	0	0	0	0	0	0	0
Mississippi	0	0	0	0	0	0	0	0	0	0
Missouri	623	465	379	339	358	495	404	489	422	390
Montana	0	0	0	0	0	0	0	0	0	0
Nebraska	278	222	62	57	40	40	53	57	61	88
Nevada	0	0	0	0	0	0	0	0	0	0
New Hampshire	23	14	29	0	0	0	0	0	0	0
New Jersey	678	630	502	440	418	525	623	708	761	758
New Mexico	0	0	0	0	0	0	0	0	0	0
New York	629	523	326	219	262	335	371	177	198	194
North Carolina	182	131	88	66	119	197	230	226	229	220
North Dakota	140	51	0	0	0	0	0	0	0	0
Ohio	1,268	1,103	687	557	555	614	753	730	691	668
Oklahoma	0	0	0	0	0	0	0	0	0	0
Oregon	0	0	0	0	0	0	0	0	0	0
Pennsylvania	1,881	1,581	1,370	1,118	1,227	1,419	1,552	1,674	1,649	1,640
Rhode Island	65	41	42	25	26	16	22	31	30	27
South Carolina	12	6	0	0	0	0	0	0	0	0
South Dakota	44	28	17	17	20	18	0	0	0	0
Tennessee	459	384	209	136	119	152	233	254	311	380
Texas	109	102	108	109	147	158	205	202	194	208
Utah	0	0	0	0	0	0	0	0	0	0
Vermont	0	0	0	0	0	0	0	0	0	0
Virginia	279	228	184	155	201	219	267	301	388	371
Washington	0	0	0	0	0	0	0	0	0	0
West Virginia	102	86	51	82	81	77	70	69	70	72
Wisconsin	140	82	44	18	26	38	32	42	40	48
Wyoming	0	0	0	0	0	0	0	0	0	0
American Samoa	0	0	0	0	0	0	0	0	0	0
Guam	0	0	0	0	0	0	0	0	0	0
Puerto Rico	0	0	0	0	0	0	0	0	0	0
Virgin Islands	0	0	0	0	0	0	0	0	0	0

[1] National and regional totals exclude American Samoa, Guam, Puerto Rico, and the Virgin Islands.

Table 32
BASIC AND RN STUDENT GRADUATIONS FROM BACCALAUREATE NURSING PROGRAMS:
1985-86 TO 1994-95[1]

| YEAR | GRADUATIONS FROM BACCALAUREATE NURSING PROGRAMS | | | |
| | Total Graduations | Basic Programs | | BRN* Programs |
		Basic Students	RN Students	RN Students
1985-86	35,550	25,170	5,698	4,682
1986-87	34,475	23,761	6,591	4,123
1987-88	32,672	21,504	6,710	4,458
1988-89	30,543	18,997	7,195	4,351
1989-90	30,763	18,571	7,241	4,951
1990-91	29,438	19,264	7,027	3,147
1991-92	32,029	21,415	7,064	3,550
1992-93	34,504	24,442	6,360	3,702
1993-94	39,693	28,912	7,018	3,763
1994-95	43,249	31,254	7,296	4,699

[1] Excludes American Samoa, Guam, Puerto Rico, and the Virgin Islands.
* BRN programs are baccalaureate programs that admit only RNs.

Table 33
GRADUATIONS OF REGISTERED NURSES FROM BACCALAUREATE NURSING PROGRAMS,
BY PREVIOUS BASIC NURSING EDUCATION AND REGION: 1990-91 TO 1994-95[1]

| YEAR AND REGION | BACCALAUREATE PROGRAMS ACCEPTING RNs | PREVIOUS NURSING CREDENTIAL[2] | | |
		Total	Diploma	Associate Degree
1990-91 (Total)	**667**	**10,174**	**3,679**	**6,495**
North Atlantic	159	2,886	1,179	1,707
Midwest	213	3,054	1,415	1,639
South	215	2,855	770	2,085
West	80	1,379	315	1,064
1991-92 (Total)	**637**	**10,614**	**3,691**	**6,923**
North Atlantic	158	2,963	1,289	1,674
Midwest	197	3,282	1,298	1,984
South	205	2,926	808	2,118
West	77	1,443	296	1,147
1992-93 (Total)	**644**	**10,062**	**3,083**	**6,979**
North Atlantic	164	2,741	1,114	1,627
Midwest	201	2,924	1,062	1,862
South	206	2,711	627	2,084
West	73	1,686	280	1,406
1993-94 (Total)	**646**	**10,781**	**3,792**	**6,989**
North Atlantic	166	3,160	1,377	1,783
Midwest	200	3,133	1,400	1,733
South	207	3,075	760	2,315
West	73	1,413	255	1,158
1994-95 (Total)	**665**	**11,995**	**3,745**	**8,250**
North Atlantic	168	3,398	1,333	2,065
Midwest	206	3,455	1,194	2,261
South	216	3,403	647	2,756
West	75	1,739	571	1,168

[1] Excludes American Samoa, Guam, Puerto Rico, and the Virgin Islands.
[2] Includes RNs in basic programs, RNs in BRN programs, and basic BSN students.

Table 34
TOTAL GRADUATIONS FROM BACCALAUREATE NURSING PROGRAMS, BY NLN REGION AND STATE:
1991 TO 1995[1]

NLN REGION AND STATE	GRADUATIONS FROM BACCALAUREATE NURSING PROGRAMS [2]									
	1991		1992		1993		1994		1995	
	Total	RNs Only	Total	RNs Only	Total	RNs Only	Total	RNs Only	Total	RNs Only
United States	**29,438**	**10,174**	**32,029**	**10,614**	**34,504**	**10,062**	**39,693**	**10,781**	**43,249**	**11,995**
North Atlantic	6,887	2,886	7,257	2,963	7,700	2,741	8,953	3,160	9,954	3,398
Midwest	8,915	3,054	9,805	3,282	10,288	2,924	11,989	3,133	13,201	3,455
South	9,376	2,855	10,496	2,926	11,505	2,711	13,508	3,075	14,436	3,403
West	4,260	1,379	4,471	1,443	5,011	1,686	5,243	1,413	5,658	1,739
Alabama	720	239	773	251	751	198	1,141	229	1,267	264
Alaska	37	16	44	12	59	11	51	5	51	4
Arizona	556	355	388	202	546	305	587	318	769	452
Arkansas	225	40	274	33	297	41	357	60	415	83
California	1,629	408	1,789	605	1,988	703	1,796	296	2,210	695
Colorado	428	131	497	133	614	200	596	135	523	104
Connecticut	332	118	422	135	424	146	464	172	618	236
Delaware	122	55	144	54	181	96	214	93	286	125
District of Columbia	158	33	216	46	175	20	237	37	236	24
Florida	929	429	1,044	425	1,107	383	1,177	482	1,179	380
Georgia	627	174	649	166	756	174	1,003	226	1,141	300
Hawaii	215	81	174	108	168	72	157	59	184	63
Idaho	117	46	103	23	130	56	127	54	109	25
Illinois	1,397	556	1,322	430	1,478	459	1,745	400	1,881	437
Indiana	897	265	1,020	298	1,018	222	1,291	316	1,742	362
Iowa	396	157	461	190	443	139	481	157	609	213
Kansas	541	155	521	126	639	103	705	115	705	68
Kentucky	489	181	541	182	581	117	658	105	639	138
Louisiana	693	85	692	91	898	80	960	88	1,031	94
Maine	158	18	201	36	230	32	288	36	323	53
Maryland	512	234	671	315	664	274	795	263	747	188
Massachusetts	925	394	961	370	988	304	1,203	392	1,141	386
Michigan	1,192	439	1,357	556	1,537	568	1,412	479	1,646	637
Minnesota	529	140	599	172	710	170	831	253	712	190
Mississippi	392	70	455	60	502	77	574	67	660	104
Missouri	639	306	812	353	921	346	1,157	447	1,365	515
Montana	106	6	154	14	120	11	164	12	179	14
Nebraska	401	142	525	158	490	99	643	95	746	104
Nevada	93	32	104	15	116	17	117	19	133	22
New Hampshire	113	32	111	34	176	57	184	64	208	84
New Jersey	570	276	515	250	572	233	664	273	641	280
New Mexico	113	67	119	60	149	80	184	91	199	106
New York	2,160	1,068	2,164	1,033	2,372	1,067	2,687	1,059	3,163	1,227
North Carolina	655	205	865	279	988	286	1,088	364	1,094	315
North Dakota	262	47	305	34	334	46	354	60	346	46
Ohio	1,540	537	1,603	591	1,636	520	2,050	573	2,030	572
Oklahoma	436	120	427	89	499	83	498	59	491	80
Oregon	285	64	328	58	295	11	345	63	385	71
Pennsylvania	2,107	818	2,289	931	2,268	712	2,605	908	2,974	892
Rhode Island	160	40	170	47	234	50	324	93	263	39
South Carolina	411	134	324	77	452	124	476	101	545	115
South Dakota	231	46	293	69	174	57	252	53	249	63
Tennessee	605	200	801	249	934	244	1,067	223	1,304	274
Texas	1,681	413	1,889	385	2,051	354	2,401	435	2,413	456
Utah	223	53	247	72	262	74	345	109	332	90
Vermont	82	34	64	27	80	24	83	33	101	52
Virginia	708	244	789	248	758	225	914	279	1,018	430
Washington	418	113	454	122	505	142	716	249	528	89
West Virginia	293	87	302	76	267	51	399	94	492	182
Wisconsin	890	264	987	305	908	195	1,068	185	1,170	248
Wyoming	40	7	70	19	59	4	58	3	56	4
American Samoa	0	0	0	0	0	0	0	0	0	0
Guam	5	5	0	0	14	7	16	0	14	3
Puerto Rico	678	151	598	133	620	208	572	134	642	79
Virgin Islands	7	1	7	1	6	2	11	6	9	1

[1] National and regional totals exclude American Samoa, Guam, Puerto Rico, and the Virgin Islands.
[2] Totals include RNs in basic programs, RNs in BRN programs, and basic BSN students.

Table 35
APPLICATIONS PER FALL ADMISSION
FOR BASIC RN PROGRAMS, BY TYPE
OF PROGRAM AND NLN REGION: 1995

NLN REGION	NUMBER OF APPLICATIONS	NUMBER OF FALL ADMISSIONS	APPLICATIONS PER FALL ADMISSIONS
ALL REPORTING RN PROGRAMS[2]			
All Regions	217,895	79,208	2.75
North Atlantic	61,056	19,722	3.10
Midwest	53,310	21,890	2.44
South	76,728	28,198	2.72
West	26,801	9,398	2.85
BACCALAUREATE PROGRAMS			
All Regions	75,194	27,241	2.76
North Atlantic	22,333	6,326	3.53
Midwest	20,776	8,777	2.37
South	22,964	8,674	2.65
West	9,121	3,464	2.63
ASSOCIATE DEGREE PROGRAMS			
All Regions	129,786	47,271	2.75
North Atlantic	31,967	11,015	2.90
Midwest	29,181	11,778	2.48
South	51,213	18,558	2.76
West	17,425	5,920	2.94
DIPLOMA PROGRAMS			
All Regions	12,915	4,696	2.75
North Atlantic	6,756	2,381	2.84
Midwest	3,353	1,335	2.51
South	2,551	966	2.64
West	255	14	18.21

[1] Excludes American Samoa, Guam, Puerto Rico and the Virgin Islands.
[2] To be included in this tabulation, a nursing program must have answered the question on number of applications and must have admitted a class in the fall of the survey year.

Table 36
PERCENTAGE OF APPLICATIONS FOR
ADMISSION ACCEPTED AND NOT ACCEPTED AND
PERCENTAGE ON WAITING LISTS FOR ALL BASIC
RN PROGRAMS, BY TYPE OF PROGRAM: 1995

ALL REPORTING RN PROGRAMS	
Total applications	100.0
Accepted	47.4
Not accepted	52.6
Percent of qualified applicants not accepted and placed on waiting lists.	14.1
BACCALAUREATE PROGRAMS	
Total applications	100.0
Accepted	54.7
Not accepted	45.3
Percent of qualified applicants not accepted and placed on waiting lists.	8.4
ASSOCIATE DEGREE PROGRAMS	
Total applications	100.0
Accepted	42.3
Not accepted	57.7
Percent of qualified applicants not accepted and placed on waiting lists.	18.3
DIPLOMA PROGRAMS	
Total applications	100.0
Accepted	54.6
Not accepted	45.4
Percent of qualified applicants not accepted and placed on waiting lists.	6.6

Section 1-4
Numeric Tables
on Male and Minority Students

Table 1
ESTIMATED NUMBER OF STUDENT ADMISSIONS
TO ALL BASIC RN PROGRAMS, BY RACE/ETHNICITY, NLN REGION AND STATE: 1994–1995[1]

NLN REGION AND STATE	NUMBER OF PROGRAMS	TOTAL NUMBER OF ADMISSIONS[2]	NUMBER OF ADMISSIONS				
			White	Black	Hispanic	Asian	American Indian
United States	**1,516**	**127,184**	**104,585**	**11,779**	**4,518**	**5,285**	**997**
North Atlantic	331	32,757	26,043	4,042	1,113	1,343	211
Midwest	441	34,225	30,396	2,080	590	942	211
South	516	45,311	37,710	4,869	1,478	942	307
West	228	14,891	10,436	788	1,337	2,058	268
Alabama	36	3,718	3,067	588	16	34	11
Alaska	2	108	90	5	4	6	3
Arizona	17	1,369	1,202	25	86	31	24
Arkansas	22	1,500	1,298	161	14	15	12
California	96	6,998	3,868	622	836	1,587	87
Colorado	17	1,098	905	50	97	31	15
Connecticut	17	1,291	1,110	100	37	39	5
Delaware	7	561	365	177	6	11	2
District of Columbia	5	373	260	66	12	31	5
Florida	40	5,173	4,082	596	321	143	32
Georgia	33	3,298	2,758	464	31	44	2
Hawaii	7	337	120	5	3	205	2
Idaho	8	330	308	0	7	8	7
Illinois	73	6,316	4,842	761	235	460	17
Indiana	46	3,404	3,173	146	43	28	13
Iowa	42	2,279	2,179	29	34	28	6
Kansas	30	1,565	1,403	77	43	25	19
Kentucky	35	2,596	2,510	64	1	14	6
Louisiana	23	2,984	2,424	471	42	37	10
Maine	15	820	797	2	4	8	7
Maryland	23	2,070	1,633	307	30	94	7
Massachusetts	44	3,277	2,754	310	109	99	4
Michigan	49	4,120	3,475	409	74	114	46
Minnesota	21	1,915	1,763	54	20	61	16
Mississippi	23	2,117	1,844	259	6	6	2
Missouri	48	3,572	3,268	216	30	48	11
Montana	5	369	326	5	5	3	29
Nebraska	14	1,000	931	24	15	28	3
Nevada	6	300	264	12	7	16	1
New Hampshire	9	615	602	7	1	4	1
New Jersey	38	3,173	2,276	435	171	278	14
New Mexico	15	705	447	12	184	12	50
New York	100	14,570	10,493	2,527	663	741	142
North Carolina	62	3,817	3,190	487	40	49	48
North Dakota	7	312	294	2	3	1	12
Ohio	69	6,367	5,883	302	55	101	27
Oklahoma	28	1,712	1,442	79	33	40	121
Oregon	16	838	740	10	29	43	14
Pennsylvania	84	7,173	6,564	381	91	113	24
Rhode Island	7	662	594	30	16	16	6
South Carolina	21	1,703	1,398	270	18	16	1
South Dakota	10	535	504	1	2	4	24
Tennessee	36	3,250	2,877	321	10	36	6
Texas	77	7,282	5,503	537	882	317	41
Utah	7	666	637	1	12	12	4
Vermont	5	242	228	7	3	3	1
Virginia	37	2,975	2,596	251	30	93	4
Washington	24	1,486	1,258	40	54	103	31
West Virginia	20	1,116	1,088	14	4	4	4
Wisconsin	32	2,840	2,681	59	36	44	17
Wyoming	8	287	271	1	13	1	1

[1] Excludes American Samoa, Guam, Puerto Rico, and the Virgin Islands.
[2] Due to rounding, the racial/ethnic estimations sometimes add up to slightly less than the true total.

Table 2
ESTIMATED NUMBER OF STUDENTS ADMISSIONS TO BASIC BACCALAUREATE
NURSING PROGRAMS, BY RACE/ETHNICITY, NLN REGION AND STATE: 1994-1995[1]

NLN REGION AND STATE	NUMBER OF PROGRAMS	TOTAL NUMBER OF ADMISSIONS[2]	NUMBER OF ADMISSIONS				
			White	Black	Hispanic	Asian	American Indian
United States	**521**	**43,451**	**35,416**	**3,780**	**1,600**	**2,376**	**271**
North Atlantic	115	9,673	7,695	1,139	346	462	30
Midwest	164	13,346	11,725	682	298	560	76
South	181	15,167	12,315	1,789	566	414	83
West	61	5,265	3,681	170	390	940	82
Alabama	13	1,143	926	177	12	23	4
Alaska	1	80	65	5	3	5	2
Arizona	4	452	380	8	36	11	17
Arkansas	9	478	423	40	8	4	3
California	24	2,298	1,248	90	221	723	16
Colorado	7	575	469	33	37	24	12
Connecticut	8	650	570	44	10	26	0
Delaware	2	283	119	153	2	8	1
District of Columbia	4	311	210	60	9	29	4
Florida	13	1,010	660	190	121	35	4
Georgia	13	1,063	891	133	11	27	1
Hawaii	3	143	53	1	2	84	2
Idaho	3	90	78	0	4	3	5
Illinois	27	2,653	2,018	244	119	263	9
Indiana	20	1,455	1,358	52	19	19	6
Iowa	12	512	481	7	11	12	0
Kansas	11	664	582	36	15	19	13
Kentucky	10	811	783	22	1	5	0
Louisiana	13	1,978	1,523	398	23	27	7
Maine	7	425	408	1	2	8	5
Maryland	7	742	558	125	16	44	2
Massachusetts	16	1,171	961	109	53	47	1
Michigan	15	1,304	1,037	117	44	87	17
Minnesota	9	725	673	8	6	34	3
Mississippi	7	623	558	60	3	1	1
Missouri	17	1,537	1,426	63	20	26	2
Montana	2	235	217	5	5	3	4
Nebraska	6	644	589	18	13	21	3
Nevada	2	111	85	6	7	12	1
New Hampshire	3	152	147	2	1	2	0
New Jersey	8	478	260	116	53	49	0
New Mexico	2	160	101	5	41	5	8
New York	32	3,157	2,294	480	158	210	14
North Carolina	12	1,049	772	241	12	18	5
North Dakota	7	312	294	2	3	1	12
Ohio	22	1,966	1,798	100	19	45	4
Oklahoma	11	560	450	33	14	23	40
Oregon	3	318	278	4	8	22	6
Pennsylvania	31	2,730	2,443	159	51	72	5
Rhode Island	3	248	216	14	7	11	0
South Carolina	8	428	364	51	2	10	1
South Dakota	4	221	218	0	1	1	1
Tennessee	18	1,341	1,218	101	2	16	4
Texas	26	2,528	1,900	157	326	136	9
Utah	3	269	253	1	9	5	1
Vermont	1	68	67	1	0	0	0
Virginia	12	958	845	57	12	43	0
Washington	6	469	393	12	13	43	8
West Virginia	9	455	444	4	3	2	2
Wisconsin	14	1,353	1,251	35	28	32	6
Wyoming	1	65	61	0	4	0	0

[1] Excludes American Samoa, Guam, Puerto Rico, and the Virgin Islands.
[2] Due to rounding, the racial/ethnic estimations sometimes add up to slightly less than the true total.

Table 3
ESTIMATED NUMBER OF STUDENT ADMISSIONS TO ASSOCIATE DEGREE NURSING PROGRAMS, BY RACE/ETHNICITY, NLN REGION AND STATE: 1994–1995[1]

NLN REGION AND STATE	NUMBER OF PROGRAMS	TOTAL NUMBER OF ADMISSIONS[2]	NUMBER OF ADMISSIONS				
			White	Black	Hispanic	Asian	American Indian
United States	**876**	**76,016**	**62,481**	**7,487**	**2,671**	**2,666**	**700**
North Atlantic	153	19,206	15,038	2,637	646	716	166
Midwest	246	18,952	16,900	1,318	265	339	129
South	311	28,391	23,914	2,918	835	500	219
West	166	9,467	6,629	614	925	1,111	186
Alabama	23	2,575	2,141	411	4	11	7
Alaska	1	28	25	0	1	1	1
Arizona	13	917	822	17	50	20	7
Arkansas	11	773	655	98	4	10	6
California	71	4,541	2,494	528	593	857	71
Colorado	10	523	436	17	60	7	3
Connecticut	6	467	390	41	22	9	5
Delaware	4	249	220	22	4	2	1
District of Columbia	1	62	50	6	3	2	1
Florida	26	4,074	3,384	395	162	106	28
Georgia	20	2,235	1,867	331	20	17	1
Hawaii	4	194	67	4	1	121	0
Idaho	5	240	230	0	3	5	2
Illinois	42	3,459	2,663	501	107	180	7
Indiana	25	1,921	1,790	92	23	9	7
Iowa	25	1,499	1,443	19	18	11	6
Kansas	19	901	821	41	28	6	6
Kentucky	25	1,785	1,727	42	0	9	6
Louisiana	9	963	860	72	19	9	3
Maine	8	395	389	1	2	0	2
Maryland	14	1,265	1,024	170	14	50	5
Massachusetts	21	1,659	1,378	182	49	48	2
Michigan	32	2,692	2,324	284	28	27	29
Minnesota	12	1,190	1,090	46	14	27	13
Mississippi	16	1,494	1,286	199	3	5	1
Missouri	27	1,725	1,547	142	10	18	9
Montana	3	134	109	0	0	0	25
Nebraska	7	260	250	5	0	6	0
Nevada	4	189	179	6	0	4	0
New Hampshire	6	463	455	5	0	2	1
New Jersey	14	1,595	1,275	173	42	99	7
New Mexico	13	545	346	7	143	7	42
New York	63	11,116	7,940	2,032	497	516	128
North Carolina	47	2,541	2,214	231	24	27	43
North Dakota	0	0	0	0	0	0	0
Ohio	34	3,574	3,313	169	31	43	19
Oklahoma	17	1,152	992	46	19	17	81
Oregon	13	520	462	6	21	21	8
Pennsylvania	23	2,663	2,453	153	15	30	12
Rhode Island	3	363	327	16	9	5	6
South Carolina	13	1,275	1,034	219	16	6	0
South Dakota	6	314	286	1	1	3	23
Tennessee	14	1,507	1,310	168	7	20	2
Texas	49	4,519	3,407	373	526	180	31
Utah	4	397	384	0	3	7	3
Vermont	4	174	161	6	3	3	1
Virginia	17	1,634	1,429	154	16	32	3
Washington	18	1,017	865	28	41	60	23
West Virginia	10	599	584	9	1	1	2
Wisconsin	17	1,417	1,373	18	5	9	10
Wyoming	7	222	210	1	9	1	1

[1] Excludes American Samoa, Guam, Puerto Rico, and the Virgin Islands.
[2] Due to rounding, the racial/ethnic estimations sometimes add up to slightly less than the true total.

55

Table 4
ESTIMATED NUMBER OF STUDENT ADMISSIONS TO DIPLOMA NURSING PROGRAMS, BY RACE/ETHNICITY, NLN REGION AND STATE: 1994–1995[1]

NLN REGION AND STATE	NUMBER OF PROGRAMS	TOTAL NUMBER OF ADMISSIONS[2]	NUMBER OF ADMISSIONS				
			White	Black	Hispanic	Asian	American Indian
United States	**119**	**7,717**	**6,688**	**512**	**247**	**243**	**26**
North Atlantic	63	3,878	3,310	266	121	165	15
Midwest	31	1,927	1,771	80	27	43	6
South	24	1,753	1,481	162	77	28	5
West	1	159	126	4	22	7	0
Alabama	0	0	0	0	0	0	0
Alaska	0	0	0	0	0	0	0
Arizona	0	0	0	0	0	0	0
Arkansas	2	249	220	23	2	1	3
California	1	159	126	4	22	7	0
Colorado	0	0	0	0	0	0	0
Connecticut	3	174	150	15	5	4	0
Delaware	1	29	26	2	0	1	0
District of Columbia	0	0	0	0	0	0	0
Florida	1	89	38	11	38	2	0
Georgia	0	0	0	0	0	0	0
Hawaii	0	0	0	0	0	0	0
Idaho	0	0	0	0	0	0	0
Illinois	4	204	161	16	9	17	1
Indiana	1	28	25	2	1	0	0
Iowa	5	268	255	3	5	5	0
Kansas	0	0	0	0	0	0	0
Kentucky	0	0	0	0	0	0	0
Louisiana	1	43	41	1	0	1	0
Maine	0	0	0	0	0	0	0
Maryland	2	63	51	12	0	0	0
Massachusetts	7	447	415	19	7	4	1
Michigan	2	124	114	8	2	0	0
Minnesota	0	0	0	0	0	0	0
Mississippi	0	0	0	0	0	0	0
Missouri	4	310	295	11	0	4	0
Montana	0	0	0	0	0	0	0
Nebraska	1	96	92	1	2	1	0
Nevada	0	0	0	0	0	0	0
New Hampshire	0	0	0	0	0	0	0
New Jersey	16	1,100	741	146	76	130	7
New Mexico	0	0	0	0	0	0	0
New York	5	297	259	15	8	15	0
North Carolina	3	227	204	15	4	4	0
North Dakota	0	0	0	0	0	0	0
Ohio	13	827	772	33	5	13	4
Oklahoma	0	0	0	0	0	0	0
Oregon	0	0	0	0	0	0	0
Pennsylvania	30	1,780	1,668	69	25	11	7
Rhode Island	1	51	51	0	0	0	0
South Carolina	0	0	0	0	0	0	0
South Dakota	0	0	0	0	0	0	0
Tennessee	4	402	349	52	1	0	0
Texas	2	235	196	7	30	1	1
Utah	0	0	0	0	0	0	0
Vermont	0	0	0	0	0	0	0
Virginia	8	383	322	40	2	18	1
Washington	0	0	0	0	0	0	0
West Virginia	1	62	60	1	0	1	0
Wisconsin	1	70	57	6	3	3	1
Wyoming	0	0	0	0	0	0	0

[1] Excludes American Samoa, Guam, Puerto Rico, and the Virgin Islands.
[2] Due to rounding, the racial/ethnic estimations sometimes add up to slightly less than the true total.

Table 5
TRENDS IN THE ESTIMATED NUMBER OF ANNUAL ADMISSIONS
OF MINORITY STUDENTS TO BASIC RN PROGRAMS, 1989–90 TO 1994–95[1]

YEAR	BLACKS		HISPANIC		ASIAN		AMERICAN INDIAN	
	Number	Percent	Number	Percent	Number	Percent	Number	Percent
ALL REPORTING RN PROGRAMS								
1989-90	12,146	11.1	3,532	3.2	3,223	3.0	704	0.6
1990-91	10,822	9.5	3,619	3.2	3,536	3.1	840	0.7
1991-92	10,476	8.5	4,258	3.5	3,972	3.2	874	0.7
1992-93	11,064	8.7	3,834	3.0	4,144	3.3	812	0.6
1993-94	11,514	8.9	4,186	3.2	4,462	3.4	959	0.7
1994-95	11,779	9.3	4,518	3.5	5,285	4.2	997	0.8
BACCALAUREATE PROGRAMS								
1989-90	3,442	11.5	881	3.0	1,117	3.7	200	0.7
1990-91	3,363	10.0	1,053	3.1	1,336	4.0	265	0.8
1991-92	3,273	8.6	1,490	3.9	1,531	4.0	283	0.7
1992-93	4,011	9.7	1,079	2.6	1,664	4.0	211	0.5
1993-94	4,005	9.3	1,312	3.0	1,738	4.0	241	0.6
1994-95	3,780	8.7	1,600	3.7	2,376	5.5	271	0.6
ASSOCIATE DEGREE PROGRAMS								
1989-90	7,756	11.3	2,426	3.5	1,807	2.6	484	0.7
1990-91	6,521	9.3	2,327	3.3	1,920	2.7	552	0.8
1991-92	6,413	8.7	2,459	3.3	2,142	2.9	568	0.8
1992-93	6,406	8.5	2,509	3.3	2,159	2.9	575	0.8
1993-94	6,867	8.9	2,645	3.4	2,461	3.2	691	0.9
1994-95	7,487	9.8	2,671	3.5	2,666	3.5	700	0.9
DIPLOMA PROGRAMS								
1989-90	945	9.4	222	2.2	298	3.0	20	0.2
1990-91	937	9.2	239	2.3	285	2.8	24	0.2
1991-92	790	7.4	309	2.9	299	2.8	23	0.2
1992-93	647	6.4	246	2.4	321	3.2	26	0.3
1993-94	642	6.7	229	2.4	263	2.7	27	0.3
1994-95	512	6.6	247	3.2	243	3.1	26	0.3

[1] Excludes American Samoa, Guam, Puerto Rico, and the Virgin Islands.

Table 6
ESTIMATED NUMBER OF STUDENT ENROLLMENTS
IN ALL BASIC RN PROGRAMS, BY RACE/ETHNICITY, NLN REGION AND STATE: 1995[1]

NLN REGION AND STATE	NUMBER OF PROGRAMS	TOTAL NUMBER OF ENROLLMENTS[2]	NUMBER OF ENROLLMENTS				
			White	Black	Hispanic	Asian	American Indian
United States	**1,516**	**261,219**	**215,197**	**24,621**	**9,039**	**10,444**	**1,900**
North Atlantic	331	75,344	61,793	8,222	2,204	2,751	374
Midwest	441	68,464	60,856	4,109	1,202	1,931	363
South	516	88,982	72,233	11,086	3,122	1,890	638
West	228	28,429	20,315	1,204	2,511	3,872	525
Alabama	36	7,637	6,060	1,397	42	89	49
Alaska	2	275	234	10	10	9	12
Arizona	17	2,363	2,041	35	189	55	44
Arkansas	22	2,880	2,573	243	16	20	26
California	96	13,074	7,624	937	1,589	2,743	181
Colorado	17	1,983	1,701	58	159	42	22
Connecticut	17	2,777	2,410	203	85	70	9
Delaware	7	1,228	892	284	14	34	4
District of Columbia	5	1,141	549	505	25	58	4
Florida	40	8,809	6,152	1,519	846	238	53
Georgia	33	5,634	4,633	815	65	115	6
Hawaii	7	992	312	19	29	628	5
Idaho	8	670	639	2	11	12	6
Illinois	73	12,388	9,639	1,298	455	971	22
Indiana	46	7,594	7,016	341	135	77	25
Iowa	42	4,004	3,872	50	33	38	8
Kansas	30	2,870	2,601	125	70	52	22
Kentucky	35	5,177	4,966	144	13	34	18
Louisiana	23	9,212	7,134	1,770	131	119	58
Maine	15	1,628	1,588	5	8	12	15
Maryland	23	3,899	3,016	662	61	141	19
Massachusetts	44	8,147	7,117	601	232	187	10
Michigan	49	8,730	7,407	865	148	232	79
Minnesota	21	3,228	2,981	100	27	91	29
Mississippi	23	3,623	3,186	399	16	16	6
Missouri	48	6,018	5,541	360	39	65	12
Montana	5	885	796	12	11	9	58
Nebraska	14	2,273	2,110	53	49	58	2
Nevada	6	534	456	14	17	37	10
New Hampshire	9	1,369	1,344	7	4	10	4
New Jersey	38	7,079	5,066	948	378	657	30
New Mexico	15	1,310	854	28	305	23	100
New York	100	33,368	25,826	4,706	1,229	1,344	262
North Carolina	62	7,135	6,210	703	70	95	55
North Dakota	7	732	681	3	5	8	35
Ohio	69	13,372	12,259	700	141	235	41
Oklahoma	28	3,130	2,621	133	66	85	223
Oregon	16	1,642	1,473	15	38	89	26
Pennsylvania	84	16,179	14,778	866	184	327	25
Rhode Island	7	1,893	1,710	89	42	42	10
South Carolina	21	3,595	3,006	502	29	52	7
South Dakota	10	1,092	1,021	7	2	10	52
Tennessee	36	6,240	5,608	515	36	69	13
Texas	77	13,496	9,910	1,316	1,649	535	83
Utah	7	1,109	1,045	3	31	20	10
Vermont	5	535	513	8	3	10	1
Virginia	37	6,236	4,935	940	74	267	18
Washington	24	3,111	2,690	68	100	203	49
West Virginia	20	2,279	2,223	28	8	15	4
Wisconsin	32	6,163	5,728	207	98	94	36
Wyoming	8	481	450	3	22	2	2

[1] Excludes American Samoa, Guam, Puerto Rico, and the Virgin Islands.
[2] Due to rounding, the racial/ethnic estimations sometimes add up to slightly less than the true total.

58

Table 7
ESTIMATED NUMBER OF STUDENT ENROLLMENTS IN BASIC BACCALAUREATE NURSING PROGRAMS, BY RACE/ETHNICITY, NLN REGION AND STATE: 1995[1]

NLN REGION AND STATE	NUMBER OF PROGRAMS	TOTAL NUMBER OF ENROLLMENTS[2]	NUMBER OF ENROLLMENTS				
			White	Black	Hispanic	Asian	American Indian
United States	**521**	**109,505**	**88,665**	**10,884**	**3,647**	**5,635**	**666**
North Atlantic	115	27,686	22,283	3,181	869	1,274	77
Midwest	164	32,714	28,739	1,877	707	1,227	164
South	181	37,018	29,059	5,505	1,192	1,027	228
West	61	12,087	8,584	321	879	2,107	197
Alabama	13	3,734	2,906	718	32	62	16
Alaska	1	220	186	9	8	7	10
Arizona	4	877	742	13	68	29	25
Arkansas	9	884	815	48	7	9	4
California	24	4,962	2,874	177	508	1,350	53
Colorado	7	1,112	966	31	64	34	17
Connecticut	8	1,534	1,375	77	35	47	0
Delaware	2	719	435	244	7	30	3
District of Columbia	4	1,045	471	496	21	54	3
Florida	13	2,436	1,341	704	301	81	8
Georgia	13	2,261	1,881	285	28	65	2
Hawaii	3	696	196	18	24	453	5
Idaho	3	217	204	0	5	5	3
Illinois	27	6,020	4,548	619	259	581	13
Indiana	20	3,685	3,390	169	75	43	8
Iowa	12	1,320	1,267	15	14	20	4
Kansas	11	1,472	1,336	63	20	42	12
Kentucky	10	1,985	1,879	75	7	18	4
Louisiana	13	6,596	4,939	1,438	87	94	38
Maine	7	1,024	991	5	4	12	12
Maryland	7	1,525	1,106	310	32	70	8
Massachusetts	16	4,003	3,585	219	101	95	3
Michigan	15	3,816	3,186	302	103	184	41
Minnesota	9	1,178	1,101	15	8	48	6
Mississippi	7	1,063	931	118	8	4	2
Missouri	17	2,897	2,688	138	33	35	3
Montana	2	670	616	12	11	9	23
Nebraska	6	1,698	1,558	43	45	50	2
Nevada	2	266	208	11	13	31	3
New Hampshire	3	530	522	0	3	5	0
New Jersey	8	1,588	975	249	145	211	7
New Mexico	2	431	284	11	101	14	21
New York	32	8,154	5,763	1,391	414	548	37
North Carolina	12	2,287	1,937	261	28	44	15
North Dakota	7	732	681	3	5	8	35
Ohio	22	5,723	5,157	355	60	138	12
Oklahoma	11	1,242	989	75	31	59	87
Oregon	3	726	634	8	17	54	13
Pennsylvania	31	7,878	7,072	447	115	237	7
Rhode Island	3	946	837	52	24	28	5
South Carolina	8	1,618	1,323	246	12	34	3
South Dakota	4	609	589	5	2	5	8
Tennessee	18	2,806	2,567	187	13	33	7
Texas	26	5,256	3,779	590	570	292	24
Utah	3	577	537	3	19	13	5
Vermont	1	265	257	1	0	7	0
Virginia	12	2,235	1,604	437	30	154	9
Washington	6	1,218	1,036	27	30	107	18
West Virginia	9	1,090	1,062	13	6	8	1
Wisconsin	14	3,564	3,238	150	83	73	20
Wyoming	1	115	101	1	11	1	1

[1] Excludes American Samoa, Guam, Puerto Rico, and the Virgin Islands.
[2] Due to rounding, the racial/ethnic estimations sometimes add up to slightly less than the true total.

Table 8
ESTIMATED NUMBER OF STUDENT ENROLLMENTS IN ASSOCIATE DEGREE
NURSING PROGRAMS, BY RACE/ETHNICITY, NLN REGION AND STATE: 1995[1]

NLN REGION AND STATE	NUMBER OF PROGRAMS	TOTAL NUMBER OF ENROLLMENTS[2]	NUMBER OF ENROLLMENTS				
			White	Black	Hispanic	Asian	American Indian
United States	**876**	**135,235**	**112,239**	**12,606**	**4,922**	**4,265**	**1,193**
North Atlantic	153	39,190	32,269	4,417	1,111	1,116	279
Midwest	246	31,644	28,350	2,049	448	603	191
South	311	48,304	40,000	5,279	1,800	822	397
West	166	16,097	11,620	861	1,563	1,724	326
Alabama	23	3,903	3,154	679	10	27	33
Alaska	1	55	48	1	2	2	2
Arizona	13	1,486	1,299	22	121	26	19
Arkansas	11	1,353	1,184	140	6	8	14
California	71	7,867	4,639	738	1,012	1,352	126
Colorado	10	871	735	27	95	8	5
Connecticut	6	966	799	99	39	20	9
Delaware	4	437	390	37	6	3	1
District of Columbia	1	96	78	9	4	4	1
Florida	26	6,247	4,761	796	491	154	45
Georgia	20	3,373	2,752	530	37	50	4
Hawaii	4	296	116	1	5	175	0
Idaho	5	453	435	2	6	7	3
Illinois	42	5,773	4,627	629	177	329	8
Indiana	25	3,709	3,443	157	58	34	17
Iowa	25	2,027	1,976	24	11	9	4
Kansas	19	1,398	1,265	62	50	10	10
Kentucky	25	3,192	3,087	69	6	16	14
Louisiana	9	2,536	2,121	329	41	25	20
Maine	8	604	597	0	4	0	3
Maryland	14	2,135	1,706	323	26	68	11
Massachusetts	21	3,058	2,540	330	111	73	4
Michigan	32	4,755	4,073	555	42	48	38
Minnesota	12	2,050	1,880	85	19	43	23
Mississippi	16	2,560	2,255	281	8	12	4
Missouri	27	2,542	2,301	200	6	25	9
Montana	3	215	180	0	0	0	35
Nebraska	7	458	439	9	2	7	0
Nevada	4	268	248	3	4	6	7
New Hampshire	6	839	822	7	1	5	4
New Jersey	14	2,709	2,110	319	95	170	16
New Mexico	13	879	570	17	204	9	79
New York	63	24,784	19,692	3,294	800	773	225
North Carolina	47	4,382	3,856	408	36	44	38
North Dakota	0	0	0	0	0	0	0
Ohio	34	5,967	5,531	274	68	75	24
Oklahoma	17	1,888	1,632	58	35	26	136
Oregon	13	916	839	7	21	35	13
Pennsylvania	23	4,584	4,214	279	30	52	10
Rhode Island	3	843	771	36	18	13	5
South Carolina	13	1,977	1,683	256	17	18	4
South Dakota	6	483	432	2	0	5	44
Tennessee	14	2,714	2,388	268	19	34	5
Texas	49	7,857	5,811	716	1,031	239	58
Utah	4	532	508	0	12	7	5
Vermont	4	270	256	7	3	3	1
Virginia	17	3,058	2,508	412	35	94	8
Washington	18	1,893	1,654	41	70	96	31
West Virginia	10	1,129	1,102	14	2	7	3
Wisconsin	17	2,482	2,383	52	15	18	14
Wyoming	7	366	349	2	11	1	1

[1] Excludes American Samoa, Guam, Puerto Rico, and the Virgin Islands.
[2] Due to rounding, the racial/ethnic estimations sometimes add up to slightly less than the true total.

60

Table 9
ESTIMATED NUMBER OF STUDENT ENROLLMENTS IN DIPLOMA
NURSING PROGRAMS, BY RACE/ETHNICITY, NLN REGION AND STATE: 1995[1]

NLN REGION AND STATE	NUMBER OF PROGRAMS	TOTAL NUMBER OF ENROLLMENTS[2]	NUMBER OF ENROLLMENTS				
			White	Black	Hispanic	Asian	American Indian
United States	**119**	**16,479**	**14,293**	**1,131**	**470**	**544**	**41**
North Atlantic	63	8,468	7,241	624	224	361	18
Midwest	31	4,106	3,767	183	47	101	8
South	24	3,660	3,174	302	130	41	13
West	1	245	111	22	69	41	2
Alabama	0	0	0	0	0	0	0
Alaska	0	0	0	0	0	0	0
Arizona	0	0	0	0	0	0	0
Arkansas	2	643	574	55	3	3	8
California	1	245	111	22	69	41	2
Colorado	0	0	0	0	0	0	0
Connecticut	3	277	236	27	11	3	0
Delaware	1	72	67	3	1	1	0
District of Columbia	0	0	0	0	0	0	0
Florida	1	126	50	19	54	3	0
Georgia	0	0	0	0	0	0	0
Hawaii	0	0	0	0	0	0	0
Idaho	0	0	0	0	0	0	0
Illinois	4	595	464	50	19	61	1
Indiana	1	200	183	15	2	0	0
Iowa	5	657	629	11	8	9	0
Kansas	0	0	0	0	0	0	0
Kentucky	0	0	0	0	0	0	0
Louisiana	1	80	74	3	3	0	0
Maine	0	0	0	0	0	0	0
Maryland	2	239	204	29	3	3	0
Massachusetts	7	1,086	992	52	20	19	3
Michigan	2	159	148	8	3	0	0
Minnesota	0	0	0	0	0	0	0
Mississippi	0	0	0	0	0	0	0
Missouri	4	579	552	22	0	5	0
Montana	0	0	0	0	0	0	0
Nebraska	1	117	113	1	2	1	0
Nevada	0	0	0	0	0	0	0
New Hampshire	0	0	0	0	0	0	0
New Jersey	16	2,782	1,981	380	138	276	7
New Mexico	0	0	0	0	0	0	0
New York	5	430	371	21	15	23	0
North Carolina	3	466	417	34	6	7	2
North Dakota	0	0	0	0	0	0	0
Ohio	13	1,682	1,571	71	13	22	5
Oklahoma	0	0	0	0	0	0	0
Oregon	0	0	0	0	0	0	0
Pennsylvania	30	3,717	3,492	140	39	38	8
Rhode Island	1	104	102	1	0	1	0
South Carolina	0	0	0	0	0	0	0
South Dakota	0	0	0	0	0	0	0
Tennessee	4	720	653	60	4	2	1
Texas	2	383	320	10	48	4	1
Utah	0	0	0	0	0	0	0
Vermont	0	0	0	0	0	0	0
Virginia	8	943	823	91	9	19	1
Washington	0	0	0	0	0	0	0
West Virginia	1	60	59	1	0	0	0
Wisconsin	1	117	107	5	0	3	2
Wyoming	0	0	0	0	0	0	0

[1] Excludes American Samoa, Guam, Puerto Rico, and the Virgin Islands.
[2] Due to rounding, the racial/ethnic estimations sometimes add up to slightly less than the true total.

Table 10
TRENDS IN THE ESTIMATED NUMBER OF ENROLLMENTS
OF MINORITY STUDENTS IN BASIC RN PROGRAMS, 1990 TO 1995[1]

YEAR	BLACKS		HISPANIC		ASIAN		AMERICAN INDIAN	
	Number	Percent	Number	Percent	Number	Percent	Number	Percent
ALL REPORTING RN PROGRAMS								
1990	23,094	10.4	6,580	3.0	6,591	3.0	1,803	0.8
1991	21,529	9.1	7,349	3.1	6,947	2.9	1,700	0.7
1992	22,147	8.6	7,667	3.0	8,306	3.2	1,685	0.6
1993	23,501	8.7	8,114	3.0	8,811	3.3	1,797	0.7
1994	24,055	9.0	8,696	3.2	9,566	3.6	1,869	0.7
1995	24,621	9.4	9,039	3.5	10,444	4.0	1,900	0.7
BACCALAUREATE PROGRAMS								
1990	9,610	11.7	2,519	3.1	3,160	3.9	586	0.7
1991	9,239	10.2	3,066	3.4	3,063	3.4	530	0.6
1992	9,154	9.0	2,896	2.8	3,966	3.9	663	0.6
1993	10,257	9.3	3,219	2.9	4,383	4.0	614	0.5
1994	10,327	9.2	3,664	3.2	4,855	4.3	698	0.6
1995	10,884	9.9	3,647	3.3	5,635	5.1	666	0.6
ASSOCIATE DEGREE PROGRAMS								
1990	11,593	9.9	3,568	3.0	2,930	2.5	1,025	0.9
1991	10,577	8.5	3,861	3.1	3,391	2.7	1,115	0.9
1992	11,327	8.5	4,237	3.2	3,687	2.8	976	0.7
1993	11,710	8.5	4,405	3.2	3,818	2.8	1,132	0.8
1994	12,397	9.1	4,478	3.3	4,093	3.0	1,123	0.8
1995	12,606	9.3	4,922	3.6	4,265	3.1	1,193	0.9
DIPLOMA PROGRAMS								
1990	1,891	8.6	491	2.2	504	2.3	190	0.9
1991	1,710	7.5	416	1.8	493	2.2	52	0.2
1992	1,666	7.2	534	2.3	653	2.8	46	0.2
1993	1,534	6.9	490	2.2	610	2.7	51	0.2
1994	1,331	6.7	554	2.8	618	3.1	48	0.2
1995	1,131	6.9	470	2.8	544	3.3	41	0.2

[1] Excludes American Samoa, Guam, Puerto Rico, and the Virgin Islands.

Table 11
ESTIMATED NUMBER OF STUDENT GRADUATIONS FROM ALL BASIC RN PROGRAMS,
BY RACE/ETHNICITY, NLN REGION AND STATE: 1994–1995[1]

NLN REGION AND STATE	NUMBER OF PROGRAMS	TOTAL NUMBER OF GRADUATIONS[2]	NUMBER OF GRADUATIONS				
			White	Black	Hispanic	Asian	American Indian
United States	**1,516**	**97,052**	**83,603**	**6,751**	**3,021**	**2,942**	**622**
North Atlantic	331	22,484	19,174	1,967	548	629	90
Midwest	441	26,865	24,705	1,268	299	469	110
South	516	35,552	30,426	3,059	1,217	592	244
West	228	12,151	9,298	457	957	1,252	178
Alabama	36	2,843	2,416	383	10	28	4
Alaska	2	74	64	1	2	2	5
Arizona	17	1,066	937	19	75	25	8
Arkansas	22	1,252	1,161	67	5	11	6
California	96	5,431	3,458	358	616	939	54
Colorado	17	877	765	25	65	10	11
Connecticut	17	896	804	52	23	13	4
Delaware	7	353	320	29	1	3	0
District of Columbia	5	246	188	35	11	11	0
Florida	40	4,285	3,364	477	321	108	15
Georgia	33	2,681	2,352	273	23	28	5
Hawaii	7	260	112	4	4	139	1
Idaho	8	312	301	1	1	6	3
Illinois	73	4,240	3,545	390	89	210	6
Indiana	46	3,232	3,029	129	34	28	8
Iowa	42	1,746	1,698	16	18	10	2
Kansas	30	1,403	1,301	45	22	23	13
Kentucky	35	2,086	2,036	32	3	10	5
Louisiana	23	1,847	1,595	193	26	21	12
Maine	15	633	621	1	6	4	1
Maryland	23	1,599	1,307	214	26	49	5
Massachusetts	44	2,604	2,341	150	73	38	2
Michigan	49	3,321	2,906	295	38	62	19
Minnesota	21	1,604	1,537	32	5	19	10
Mississippi	23	1,572	1,409	142	12	6	2
Missouri	48	2,565	2,430	95	17	15	8
Montana	5	285	264	2	2	2	15
Nebraska	14	927	871	18	18	15	3
Nevada	6	231	193	6	9	20	5
New Hampshire	9	498	491	2	2	2	1
New Jersey	38	2,319	1,801	231	111	160	16
New Mexico	15	582	398	12	124	12	36
New York	100	8,232	6,352	1,187	270	298	54
North Carolina	62	3,100	2,805	233	10	22	24
North Dakota	7	300	285	1	2	4	8
Ohio	69	4,964	4,632	228	42	53	6
Oklahoma	28	1,349	1,134	55	24	25	112
Oregon	16	795	733	6	13	29	15
Pennsylvania	84	5,936	5,558	246	36	84	9
Rhode Island	7	624	569	28	12	13	3
South Carolina	21	1,254	1,100	137	10	7	1
South Dakota	10	425	398	1	1	5	20
Tennessee	36	2,632	2,459	139	11	18	3
Texas	77	5,875	4,494	460	693	180	44
Utah	7	727	689	1	16	13	6
Vermont	5	143	129	6	3	3	0
Virginia	37	2,314	1,953	246	37	73	5
Washington	24	1,299	1,184	22	25	53	16
West Virginia	20	863	841	8	6	6	1
Wisconsin	32	2,138	2,073	18	13	25	7
Wyoming	8	212	200	0	5	2	3

[1] Excludes American Samoa, Guam, Puerto Rico, and the Virgin Islands.
[2] Due to rounding, the racial/ethnic estimations sometimes add up to slightly less than the true total.

Table 12
ESTIMATED NUMBER OF STUDENT GRADUATIONS
FROM BASIC BACCALAUREATE NURSING PROGRAMS, BY RACE/ETHNICITY, NLN REGION
AND STATE: 1994–1995[1]

NLN REGION AND STATE	NUMBER OF PROGRAMS	TOTAL NUMBER OF GRADUATIONS[2]	NUMBER OF GRADUATIONS				
			White	Black	Hispanic	Asian	American Indian
United States	**521**	**31,254**	**26,567**	**2,277**	**913**	**1,258**	**170**
North Atlantic	115	6,556	5,456	600	164	254	15
Midwest	164	9,746	8,903	410	123	264	42
South	181	11,033	9,131	1,165	388	283	68
West	61	3,919	3,077	102	238	457	45
Alabama	13	1,003	839	137	7	20	1
Alaska	1	47	39	1	1	1	5
Arizona	4	317	268	10	23	11	5
Arkansas	9	332	310	17	1	3	0
California	24	1,515	997	58	140	310	10
Colorado	7	419	381	10	18	7	3
Connecticut	8	382	353	15	4	9	1
Delaware	2	161	148	11	0	2	0
District of Columbia	4	212	159	33	10	10	0
Florida	13	799	533	132	99	35	1
Georgia	13	841	745	75	6	13	2
Hawaii	3	121	54	4	3	59	1
Idaho	3	84	78	0	1	2	3
Illinois	27	1,444	1,216	97	28	99	4
Indiana	20	1,380	1,273	65	17	23	1
Iowa	12	396	388	3	3	2	0
Kansas	11	637	584	22	7	18	6
Kentucky	10	501	483	13	1	4	0
Louisiana	13	937	793	118	11	10	5
Maine	7	270	263	1	1	4	1
Maryland	7	559	440	85	11	25	0
Massachusetts	16	755	670	41	29	15	0
Michigan	15	1,009	865	77	18	42	7
Minnesota	9	522	490	8	5	12	7
Mississippi	7	556	496	53	3	4	0
Missouri	17	850	798	34	11	5	1
Montana	2	165	159	2	2	2	0
Nebraska	6	642	598	13	15	14	2
Nevada	2	111	82	4	7	15	3
New Hampshire	3	124	123	0	0	1	0
New Jersey	8	361	264	45	17	33	2
New Mexico	2	93	62	1	20	5	5
New York	32	1,936	1,327	337	79	119	9
North Carolina	12	779	641	120	2	12	4
North Dakota	7	300	285	1	2	4	8
Ohio	22	1,458	1,350	78	9	19	1
Oklahoma	11	411	321	32	9	15	35
Oregon	3	314	284	2	8	17	3
Pennsylvania	31	2,082	1,899	105	19	55	2
Rhode Island	3	224	201	12	5	6	0
South Carolina	8	430	376	45	5	5	0
South Dakota	4	186	180	0	0	2	4
Tennessee	18	1,030	951	65	4	9	0
Texas	26	1,957	1,451	190	208	88	18
Utah	3	242	228	0	6	6	2
Vermont	1	49	49	0	0	0	0
Virginia	12	588	456	80	16	35	1
Washington	6	439	399	10	6	20	4
West Virginia	9	310	296	3	5	5	1
Wisconsin	14	922	876	12	8	24	1
Wyoming	1	52	46	0	3	2	1

[1] Excludes American Samoa, Guam, Puerto Rico, and the Virgin Islands.
[2] Due to rounding, the racial/ethnic estimations sometimes add up to slightly less than the true total.

Table 13
ESTIMATED NUMBER OF STUDENT GRADUATIONS FROM ASSOCIATE DEGREE NURSING PROGRAMS, BY RACE/ETHNICITY, NLN REGION AND STATE: 1994–1995[1]

NLN REGION AND STATE	NUMBER OF PROGRAMS	TOTAL NUMBER OF GRADUATIONS[2]	NUMBER OF GRADUATIONS				
			White	Black	Hispanic	Asian	American Indian
United States	**876**	**58,749**	**50,754**	**4,085**	**1,917**	**1,519**	**431**
North Atlantic	153	12,689	10,801	1,218	308	290	63
Midwest	246	15,243	14,058	774	154	180	67
South	311	22,748	19,747	1,758	773	284	171
West	166	8,069	6,148	335	682	765	130
Alabama	23	1,840	1,577	246	3	8	3
Alaska	1	27	25	0	1	1	0
Arizona	13	749	669	9	52	14	3
Arkansas	11	636	591	31	3	5	5
California	71	3,753	2,388	280	439	599	41
Colorado	10	458	384	15	47	3	8
Connecticut	6	346	301	27	13	3	2
Delaware	4	176	156	18	1	1	0
District of Columbia	1	34	29	2	1	1	0
Florida	26	3,391	2,783	327	197	69	14
Georgia	20	1,840	1,607	198	17	15	3
Hawaii	4	139	58	0	1	80	0
Idaho	5	228	223	1	0	4	0
Illinois	42	2,614	2,191	274	50	97	2
Indiana	25	1,767	1,675	62	16	4	7
Iowa	25	1,084	1,051	11	12	6	2
Kansas	19	766	717	23	15	5	7
Kentucky	25	1,585	1,553	19	2	6	5
Louisiana	9	875	769	73	15	11	7
Maine	8	363	358	0	5	0	0
Maryland	14	934	777	115	14	23	5
Massachusetts	21	1,413	1,270	87	38	17	1
Michigan	32	2,163	1,905	208	17	20	12
Minnesota	12	1,082	1,047	24	0	7	3
Mississippi	16	1,016	913	89	9	2	2
Missouri	27	1,325	1,258	50	5	6	7
Montana	3	120	105	0	0	0	15
Nebraska	7	197	190	2	2	1	0
Nevada	4	120	111	2	2	5	2
New Hampshire	6	374	368	2	2	1	1
New Jersey	14	1,200	970	115	39	69	7
New Mexico	13	489	336	11	104	7	31
New York	63	6,102	4,850	844	188	169	45
North Carolina	47	2,101	1,957	103	6	9	20
North Dakota	0	0	0	0	0	0	0
Ohio	34	2,838	2,657	113	31	30	5
Oklahoma	17	938	813	23	15	10	77
Oregon	13	481	449	4	5	12	12
Pennsylvania	23	2,214	2,075	102	11	21	4
Rhode Island	3	373	344	15	7	5	3
South Carolina	13	824	724	92	5	2	1
South Dakota	6	239	218	1	1	3	16
Tennessee	14	1,222	1,165	40	7	7	3
Texas	49	3,710	2,873	260	461	91	23
Utah	4	485	461	1	10	7	4
Vermont	4	94	80	6	3	3	0
Virginia	17	1,355	1,171	138	18	25	3
Washington	18	860	785	12	19	33	12
West Virginia	10	481	474	4	1	1	0
Wisconsin	17	1,168	1,149	6	5	1	6
Wyoming	7	160	154	0	2	0	2

[1] Excludes American Samoa, Guam, Puerto Rico, and the Virgin Islands.
[2] Due to rounding, the racial/ethnic estimations sometimes add up to slightly less than the true total.

TABLE 14
ESTIMATED NUMBER OF STUDENT GRADUATIONS FROM DIPLOMA NURSING PROGRAMS,
BY RACE/ETHNICITY, NLN REGION AND STATE: 1994–1995[1]

NLN REGION AND STATE	NUMBER OF PROGRAMS	TOTAL NUMBER OF GRADUATIONS[2]	NUMBER OF GRADUATIONS				
			White	Black	Hispanic	Asian	American Indian
United States	**119**	**7,049**	**6,282**	**389**	**191**	**165**	**21**
North Atlantic	63	3,239	2,917	149	76	85	12
Midwest	31	1,876	1,744	84	22	25	1
South	24	1,771	1,548	136	56	25	5
West	1	163	73	20	37	30	3
Alabama	0	0	0	0	0	0	0
Alaska	0	0	0	0	0	0	0
Arizona	0	0	0	0	0	0	0
Arkansas	2	284	260	19	1	3	1
California	1	163	73	20	37	30	3
Colorado	0	0	0	0	0	0	0
Connecticut	3	168	150	10	6	1	1
Delaware	1	16	16	0	0	0	0
District of Columbia	0	0	0	0	0	0	0
Florida	1	95	48	18	25	4	0
Georgia	0	0	0	0	0	0	0
Hawaii	0	0	0	0	0	0	0
Idaho	0	0	0	0	0	0	0
Illinois	4	182	138	19	11	14	0
Indiana	1	85	81	2	1	1	0
Iowa	5	266	259	2	3	2	0
Kansas	0	0	0	0	0	0	0
Kentucky	0	0	0	0	0	0	0
Louisiana	1	35	33	2	0	0	0
Maine	0	0	0	0	0	0	0
Maryland	2	106	90	14	1	1	0
Massachusetts	7	436	401	22	6	6	1
Michigan	2	149	136	10	3	0	0
Minnesota	0	0	0	0	0	0	0
Mississippi	0	0	0	0	0	0	0
Missouri	4	390	374	11	1	4	0
Montana	0	0	0	0	0	0	0
Nebraska	1	88	83	3	1	0	1
Nevada	0	0	0	0	0	0	0
New Hampshire	0	0	0	0	0	0	0
New Jersey	16	758	567	71	55	58	7
New Mexico	0	0	0	0	0	0	0
New York	5	194	175	6	3	10	0
North Carolina	3	220	207	10	2	1	0
North Dakota	0	0	0	0	0	0	0
Ohio	13	668	625	37	2	4	0
Oklahoma	0	0	0	0	0	0	0
Oregon	0	0	0	0	0	0	0
Pennsylvania	30	1,640	1,584	39	6	8	3
Rhode Island	1	27	24	1	0	2	0
South Carolina	0	0	0	0	0	0	0
South Dakota	0	0	0	0	0	0	0
Tennessee	4	380	343	34	0	2	0
Texas	2	208	170	10	24	1	3
Utah	0	0	0	0	0	0	0
Vermont	0	0	0	0	0	0	0
Virginia	8	371	326	28	3	13	1
Washington	0	0	0	0	0	0	0
West Virginia	1	72	71	1	0	0	0
Wisconsin	1	48	48	0	0	0	0
Wyoming	0	0	0	0	0	0	0

[1] Excludes American Samoa, Guam, Puerto Rico, and the Virgin Islands.
[2] Due to rounding, the racial/ethnic estimations sometimes add up to slightly less than the true total.

Table 15
TRENDS IN THE ESTIMATED NUMBER OF GRADUATIONS
OF MINORITY STUDENTS FROM BASIC RN PROGRAMS, 1989–90 TO 1994–95[1]

YEAR	BLACKS		HISPANIC		ASIAN		AMERICAN INDIAN	
	Number	Percent	Number	Percent	Number	Percent	Number	Percent
ALL REPORTING RN PROGRAMS								
1989-90	5,801	8.8	2,046	3.1	1,604	2.4	363	0.6
1990-91	5,350	7.4	2,026	2.8	1,809	2.5	363	0.5
1991-92	5,786	7.2	2,404	3.0	2,037	2.5	461	0.6
1992-93	6,024	6.8	2,340	2.6	2,270	2.6	610	0.7
1993-94	6,455	6.8	2,841	3.0	2,796	2.9	566	0.6
1994-95	6,751	7.0	3,021	3.1	2,942	3.0	622	0.6
BACCALAUREATE PROGRAMS								
1989-90	1,910	10.3	602	3.2	683	3.7	101	0.5
1990-91	1,552	8.0	525	2.7	765	4.0	115	0.6
1991-92	1,670	7.8	641	3.0	744	3.5	126	0.6
1992-93	1,799	7.4	587	2.4	918	3.8	193	0.8
1993-94	1,912	6.6	870	3.0	1,116	3.9	133	0.5
1994-95	2,277	7.3	913	2.9	1,258	4.0	170	0.5
ASSOCIATE DEGREE PROGRAMS								
1989-90	3,522	8.3	1,342	3.2	836	2.0	255	0.5
1990-91	3,415	7.3	1,307	2.8	937	2.0	236	0.5
1991-92	3,762	7.1	1,605	3.0	1,179	2.2	322	0.6
1992-93	3,860	6.8	1,584	2.8	1,211	2.1	405	0.7
1993-94	4,150	7.1	1,790	3.0	1,475	2.5	409	0.7
1994-95	4,085	7.0	1,917	3.3	1,519	2.6	431	0.7
DIPLOMA PROGRAMS								
1989-90	365	7.1	98	1.9	80	1.6	6	0.1
1990-91	381	6.2	196	3.2	109	1.8	11	0.2
1991-92	354	5.4	158	2.4	114	1.7	13	0.2
1992-93	365	5.3	169	2.4	141	2.0	12	0.2
1993-94	393	5.5	181	2.5	205	2.9	24	0.3
1994-95	389	5.5	191	2.7	165	2.3	21	0.3

[1] Excludes American Samoa, Guam, Puerto Rico, and the Virgin Islands.

Table 16
ADMISSIONS OF MEN TO ALL BASIC RN PROGRAMS, BY NLN REGION: 1994–1995[1]

NLN REGION	NUMBER OF PROGRAMS REPORTING	TOTAL ADMISSIONS	MEN	
			Number	Percent
ALL REPORTING RN PROGRAMS				
All Regions	**1,206**	**104,439**	**13,947**	**13.3**
North Atlantic	271	28,067	4,041	14.4
Midwest	339	27,255	2,994	11.0
South	417	36,937	5,136	13.9
West	179	12,180	1,776	14.6
BACCALAUREATE PROGRAMS				
All Regions	**404**	**35,131**	**4,486**	**12.8**
North Atlantic	89	7,684	868	11.3
Midwest	123	10,803	1,227	11.4
South	140	11,767	1,751	14.9
West	52	4,877	640	13.1
ASSOCIATE DEGREE PROGRAMS				
All Regions	**697**	**62,419**	**8,564**	**13.7**
North Atlantic	126	16,872	2,646	15.7
Midwest	189	14,626	1,557	10.6
South	255	23,618	3,225	13.7
West	127	7,303	1,136	15.6
DIPLOMA PROGRAMS				
All Regions	**105**	**6,889**	**897**	**13.0**
North Atlantic	56	3,511	527	15.0
Midwest	27	1,826	210	11.5
South	22	1,552	160	10.3
West	0	0	0	0

[1] Excludes American Samoa, Guam, Puerto Rico, and the Virgin Islands.

Table 17
TRENDS IN ADMISSIONS OF MEN TO ALL BASIC RN PROGRAMS: 1985–1995[1]

YEAR	NUMBER OF PROGRAMS REPORTING	MEN	
		Number	Percent
ALL REPORTING RN PROGRAMS			
1985	1,260	6,344	6.3
1986	1,228	5,715	6.6
1987	1,192	5,302	7.2
1988	1,257	5,958	7.3
1989	1,272	7,558	8.2
1991	1,194	10,033	10.7
1992	1,219	12,568	12.0
1993	1,243	14,111	12.9
1994	1,205	14,463	13.5
1995	1,206	13,947	13.3
BACCALAUREATE PROGRAMS			
1985	374	1,972	5.9
1986	382	1,783	6.0
1987	370	1,560	7.1
1988	412	1,675	6.7
1989	429	1,820	7.0
1991	412	3,003	10.4
1992	405	3,837	12.2
1993	412	4,434	12.6
1994	399	4,369	12.4
1995	404	4,486	12.8
ASSOCIATE DEGREE PROGRAMS			
1985	643	3,540	6.5
1986	643	3,432	7.1
1987	630	3,290	7.6
1988	682	3,726	7.6
1989	695	4,857	8.6
1991	654	6,089	10.9
1992	691	7,580	12.0
1993	711	8,357	13.1
1994	694	8,971	14.1
1995	697	8,564	13.7
DIPLOMA PROGRAMS			
1985	243	832	5.9
1986	203	498	5.3
1987	192	452	5.9
1988	163	557	6.8
1989	148	881	9.2
1991	128	941	10.1
1992	123	1,151	11.5
1993	120	1,320	13.6
1994	112	1,123	13.8
1995	105	897	13.0

[1] Excludes American Samoa, Guam, Puerto Rico, and the Virgin Islands.

Table 18
ENROLLMENTS OF MEN IN ALL BASIC RN PROGRAMS, BY NLN REGION: 1995[1]

NLN REGION	NUMBER OF PROGRAMS REPORTING	TOTAL ENROLLMENTS	MEN	
			Number	Percent
ALL REPORTING RN PROGRAMS				
All Regions	**1,240**	**222,346**	**29,061**	**13.1**
North Atlantic	273	64,328	9,611	14.9
Midwest	356	56,721	5,819	10.3
South	426	76,478	10,252	13.4
West	185	24,819	3,379	13.6
BACCALAUREATE PROGRAMS				
All Regions	**421**	**93,357**	**11,330**	**12.1**
North Atlantic	90	22,578	2,283	10.1
Midwest	132	27,411	2,983	10.9
South	145	32,004	4,606	14.4
West	54	11,364	1,458	12.8
ASSOCIATE DEGREE PROGRAMS				
All Regions	**705**	**113,385**	**15,841**	**14.0**
North Atlantic	125	34,157	6,257	18.3
Midwest	193	25,204	2,436	9.7
South	257	40,814	5,286	13.0
West	130	13,210	1,862	14.1
DIPLOMA PROGRAMS				
All Regions	**114**	**15,604**	**1,890**	**12.1**
North Atlantic	58	7,593	1,071	14.1
Midwest	31	4,106	400	9.7
South	24	3,660	360	9.8
West	1	245	59	24.1

[1] Excludes American Samoa, Guam, Puerto Rico, and the Virgin Islands.

Table 19
TRENDS IN ENROLLMENTS OF MEN IN ALL BASIC RN PROGRAMS: 1985–1995[1]

YEAR	NUMBER OF PROGRAMS REPORTING	MEN	
		Number	Percent
ALL REPORTING RN PROGRAMS			
1985	1,260	9,623	5.2
1986	1,228	8,259	4.4
1988	1,257	10,100	6.2
1989	1,272	12,404	6.9
1991	1,194	19,072	9.9
1992	1,157	22,823	11.1
1993	1,289	30,005	12.4
1994	1,236	28,875	12.6
1995	1,240	29,061	13.1
BACCALAUREATE PROGRAMS			
1985	374	3,787	4.9
1986	382	2,219	2.4
1988	412	3,363	5.4
1989	429	3,867	5.9
1991	412	6,973	9.8
1992	370	8,353	11.0
1993	438	12,470	12.3
1994	418	11,717	12.0
1995	421	11,330	12.1
ASSOCIATE DEGREE PROGRAMS			
1985	643	4,254	5.5
1986	643	4,992	6.7
1988	682	5,539	6.8
1989	695	7,033	7.5
1991	654	10,068	10.1
1992	669	12,178	11.2
1993	730	14,924	12.6
1994	700	14,705	13.2
1995	705	15,841	14.0
DIPLOMA PROGRAMS			
1985	243	1,582	5.5
1986	203	1,048	4.9
1988	163	1,198	6.5
1989	148	1,504	7.8
1991	128	2,031	9.6
1992	118	2,292	10.8
1993	121	2,611	12.2
1994	118	2,453	12.9
1995	114	1,890	12.1

[1] Excludes American Samoa, Guam, Puerto Rico, and the Virgin Islands.

Table 20
GRADUATIONS OF MEN FROM ALL BASIC RN PROGRAMS, BY NLN REGIONS: 1994–1995[1]

NLN REGION	NUMBER OF PROGRAMS REPORTING	TOTAL GRADUATIONS	MEN	
			Number	Percent
ALL REPORTING RN PROGRAMS				
All Regions	**1,171**	**81,703**	**10,140**	**12.4**
North Atlantic	266	19,208	2,420	12.6
Midwest	328	21,877	2,188	10.0
South	401	30,472	4,082	13.4
West	176	10,146	1,450	14.3
BACCALAUREATE PROGRAMS				
All Regions	**390**	**26,965**	**3,290**	**12.2**
North Atlantic	85	5,582	593	10.6
Midwest	120	8,473	903	10.7
South	133	9,227	1,277	13.8
West	52	3,683	517	14.0
ASSOCIATE DEGREE PROGRAMS				
All Regions	**672**	**48,149**	**5,991**	**12.4**
North Atlantic	124	10,708	1,421	13.3
Midwest	179	11,574	1,074	9.3
South	246	19,567	2,619	13.4
West	123	6,300	877	13.9
DIPLOMA PROGRAMS				
All Regions	**109**	**6,589**	**859**	**13.0**
North Atlantic	57	2,918	406	13.9
Midwest	29	1,830	211	11.5
South	22	1,678	186	11.1
West	1	163	56	34.4

[1] Excludes American Samoa, Guam, Puerto Rico, and the Virgin Islands.

Table 21
TRENDS IN GRADUATIONS OF MEN FROM ALL BASIC RN PROGRAMS: 1985–1995[1]

YEAR	NUMBER OF PROGRAMS REPORTING	MEN	
		Number	Percent
ALL REPORTING RN PROGRAMS			
1985	1,260	3,908	5.7
1986	1,228	3,916	5.5
1988	1,237	3,264	5.7
1989	1,272	3,080	5.7
1991	1,194	4,745	8.4
1992	1,006	6,178	9.9
1993	1,167	7,808	10.5
1994	1,178	9,130	11.4
1995	1,171	10,140	12.4
BACCALAUREATE PROGRAMS			
1985	374	1,198	5.6
1986	382	1,146	4.3
1988	393	983	5.2
1989	429	851	5.0
1991	412	1,201	8.2
1992	298	1,639	10.4
1993	376	2,233	10.5
1994	393	2,816	11.1
1995	390	3,290	12.2
ASSOCIATE DEGREE PROGRAMS			
1985	643	2,201	6.1
1986	643	2,326	6.8
1988	681	1,896	5.9
1989	695	1,989	6.0
1991	654	3,106	8.5
1992	609	4,027	9.7
1993	679	4,897	10.4
1994	672	5,509	11.5
1995	672	5,991	12.4
DIPLOMA PROGRAMS			
1985	243	509	4.5
1986	203	444	4.4
1988	163	385	6.7
1989	148	240	5.2
1991	128	438	8.0
1992	99	512	9.7
1993	112	678	10.6
1994	113	805	12.0
1995	109	859	13.0

[1] Excludes American Samoa, Guam, Puerto Rico, and the Virgin Islands.

PART TWO
LEADERS IN THE MAKING:
GRADUATE EDUCATION IN NURSING

Section 2-1
Executive Summary

EXECUTIVE SUMMARY

TRENDS IN MASTER'S NURSING EDUCATION

The 1995 NLN Annual Survey of Graduate Nursing Education showed growth in programs, enrollment and graduation. In keeping with the recent proliferation of master's degree programs, 30 new master's programs were established in 1995, the largest increase in more than 10 years. Master's degree programs now total 306 programs (Figure 1). Nursing is a nation wide phenomenon, but programs vary widely by geographic location. The highest number of programs was located in the South at 94 and the lowest number of programs was located in the West at 47. States such as New York (26) and Pennsylvania (25) continue to have the most programs.

Increasingly, more nurses are prepared at the master's level. Enrollments in 1995 continued an upward trend, reaching 35,707 (Figure 2). Part-time enrollments continued to be the norm for students attending master's programs; however full-time enrollments were on the rise (29.6%).

The results of the survey revealed that the number of students graduating from master's programs continued to increase, with a total of 9,261 graduates reported for the 1994-95 academic year (Figure 3). An examination by geographic region showed that the highest number of graduates was from the South (31.8%) and the lowest was from the West (17.7%).

TRENDS IN DOCTORAL EDUCATION

The last decade has brought significant change in doctoral education. For the second consecutive year there was an increase in doctoral nursing programs. In 1995 the number of doctoral programs was 64 (Figure 4), an increase of four new programs from the previous year.

There was also a rise in doctoral enrollment (Figure 5), reaching a total of 3,230 students in 1995. Part-time attendance remained the main avenue for doctoral students but full-time attendance showed a small increase of 2 percent.

Since 1991-92 we have seen a two-year decline in the number of graduates from doctoral programs. For the first time since then there was a reported increase in graduations from doctoral programs, with a reported 425 new graduates for the 1994-95 academic year (Figure 6). This increase has only begun to parallel the increase in the total enrollment.

MINORITIES IN GRADUATE NURSING EDUCATION

With respect to minority students, the overall results from the survey were consistent with those from previous years. The gap between minority and white enrollments and graduations have not narrowed. The stagnation in minority representation occurred despite a steady increase in the number of total enrollments. Minority enrollment in graduate nursing programs has consistently represented a small segment of the total enrollment pool. Total enrollment of all minority groups fell from 13.7 percent in 1994 to 13.2 percent in 1995 (Figure 12). Across ethnicity, blacks continue to represent the greatest portion of the minority population (6.3 percent) followed by Asians (3.7 percent), Hispanics (2.7 percent) and American Indians (0.5 percent).

Concurrent with enrollment of minorities, graduations of minorities decreased by 0.8 percent in 1995 (Figure 13). The largest group of minority graduates was blacks at 5.6 percent and the smallest group was American-Indians at 0.6 percent. Blacks and Hispanics showed a decrease in the number of graduates whereas Asians and American Indians showed an increase.

MEN IN GRADUATE NURSING EDUCATION

Enrollment of men remained virtually unchanged from the previous year, representing 5.9 percent of the total enrollment. The majority of male students (Figure 14) were located in the West (7.4 percent) and the fewest in the Midwest (4.6 percent). Male graduates comprised 6.2 percent of the total graduating class, down by 1.5 percent from 1995.

SPECIALTY AREAS IN ADVANCED NURSING

With the increase of master's programs also came an increasing number of new specialties and programs offering these specialties. There is a myriad of different subspecialties, preparing master's degree nurses for roles in several different fields. These include working in health care and academic settings, assuming roles in research, education, administration and acting as primary health care providers. The recent trends in health care, particularly the demand for various health services, especially community-based care, have been important factors in determining which nursing specialties are selected over others. In 1995 nurse practitioner programs continued to represent the highest rates of enrollment, accounting for 52.3 percent of all students (Figure 9) compared to advanced clinical practice at 28.4 percent followed by administration-management at 11 percent and teaching at 8.3 percent.

More graduate nursing schools offered nurse practitioner specialties, increasing from 193 programs in 1994 to 199 programs in 1995 (Figure 10). Among specialties within nurse practitioner programs, family practice nursing was offered more often than any other field followed by adult nursing and pediatric nursing. School practice nursing was offered least often by nurse practitioner programs.

Within advanced clinical practice, students selected adult health/medical-surgical nursing (Figure 11) most often, followed by community/public health and psychiatric-mental health. Oncology was the least chosen area of study.

RESULTS FROM SUPPLEMENTARY QUESTIONS IN THE ANNUAL SURVEY

Several supplementary questions were included in the 1995 NLN Annual Survey to reflect current issues facing nursing education. These questions addressed topics including involvement in international education, interdisciplinary activities, clinical experience, the use of computers and the plan to reduce the number of students admitted.

Graduate nursing programs reported having multiple and diverse relationships with several organizations at the international level. Close to 20 percent of master's programs reported having some type of faculty-to-faculty exchange (Figure 7) and close to a third of the schools indicated that they had either a study abroad program for students or collaborative research/teaching/ training program with international agencies or universities. Collaborative agreement through non-governmental organizations (NGO) was uncommon. In comparison, doctoral programs overall had a higher percentage of schools reporting involvement in all categories of international academic activities than the master's programs.

Most programs had faculty engaged in interdisciplinary activities. More than 75 percent of the master's programs had faculty involved in teaching interdisciplinary courses and preparing research grants with faculty from other disciplines (Figure 8). More than 50 percent were involved in developing interdisciplinary faculty practice and serving on dissertation committees for students from other disciplines. However, only 38 percent participated in the regional accreditation of colleges. Doctoral programs reported a higher percentage of faculty involvement in all interdisciplinary activities than master's programs.

Master's programs selected community-based care settings most often as the site for nursing students' clinical experience (40 percent) followed by acute (21.9 percent) and long-term care settings (8.1 percent). Less than 10 percent of all doctoral programs used any type of clinical setting as areas where doctoral students spent time obtaining clinical experience.

Only 5.3 percent of master's programs planned any reductions in student admissions. The reasons given most often for reducing the number of students admitted were, perceived lack of jobs (8.1 percent), lack of qualified applicants (4.6 percent) and budget reductions (3.5 percent). The average estimated percentage of the reduction was less than 20 percent. Less than 15 percent of the doctoral programs reported that they intended to reduce the number of students admitted to the program. These programs plan to reduce admission by less than 1 percent.

CURRENT ISSUES IN NURSING

Our population is changing at a rapid rate due to external and internal social factors that influence the profile of the country. Nursing is facing a major dilemma when attempting to prepare their students for this emerging population and therefore needs to accommodate the necessary changes ahead in terms of curriculum and its cognitive mind set. As populations change so should the policies of nursing institutions to meet the changing needs of the people they serve—if they do not they will surely wither and die.

If nursing programs do not recruit students and expose them to the different settings that fit the new demographic they will be graduating nurses with no place to go. Nursing must recognize the link between population and nursing. The Pew Commission reports that health care professions must be more sensitive culturally in meeting the needs of an ever increasing diverse health care population.[1] It is imperative that nursing programs examine the needs of the population and use these findings to design their curriculum.

There is a great demand for comparative data systems on nurse staffing and recruitment. This will enable us as health care providers, educators and policy makers to make predictions and projections to avoid the shortages that the nursing community has previously experienced. Policy makers look to trends in nursing employment as a sign of change in health care. This can also be a predictor of factors that will affect the composition of nursing staff in the future. Other measures that must continually be analyzed are patient outcomes and cost effectiveness within the health care system.

Changes are made within the health care system without appropriate evaluation of the supply of nurses. The health care community should utilize more fully the widespread availability of information on nursing. Included in this databank should be statistical information regarding practicing nurses, their specialties and sub-specialties, where the demand and supply for nurses are geographically located and a general profile of the nursing community. In addition, other useful data that should be available is salary information, hospital departments in which nurses are working and the overall trends in the workplace. Rather than preparing an indeterminate number of nurses, the nursing community needs to take full advantage of the technology currently available. This would enable us to avoid the imbalance of supply and demand of registered nurses that has been experienced in the past. We at the National League for Nursing have already taken the initiative and begun to compile such a large scale database that is available to professionals and the general public.

Delroy Louden, PhD
Executive Director
NLN Center for Research in Nursing
   Education and Community Health

Sherlene Trotman, MS
Research Coordinator
NLN Center for Research in Nursing
   Education and Community Health

REFERENCES

1. Pew Health Commission Report, 1995. Critical Challenges: Revitalizing the Health Professions for the 21st Century. San Francisco, Pew Charitable Trust.

Section 2-2
Graphs

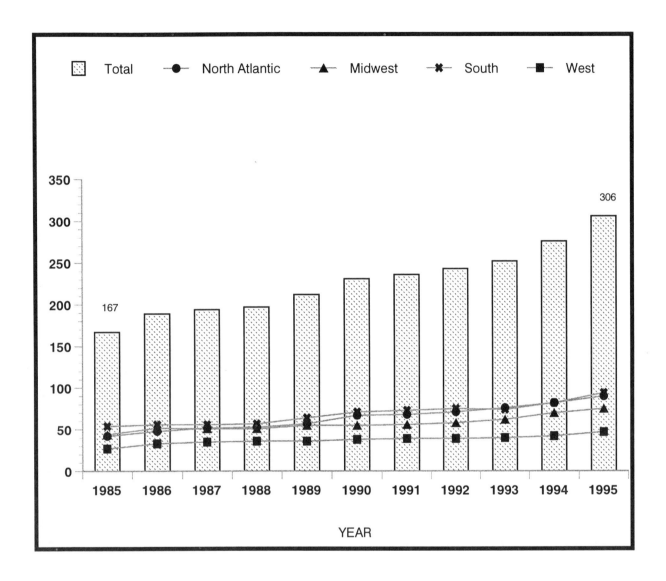

Figure 1. Number Of Master's Programs Reached 306

Thirty new master's programs opened in 1995 to reach a total of 306 programs. New programs were introduced in all regions of the United States. The South had the highest number of programs at 94, followed by the North Atlantic (90) and the Midwest (75). The lowest number of programs continue to be in the West at 47.

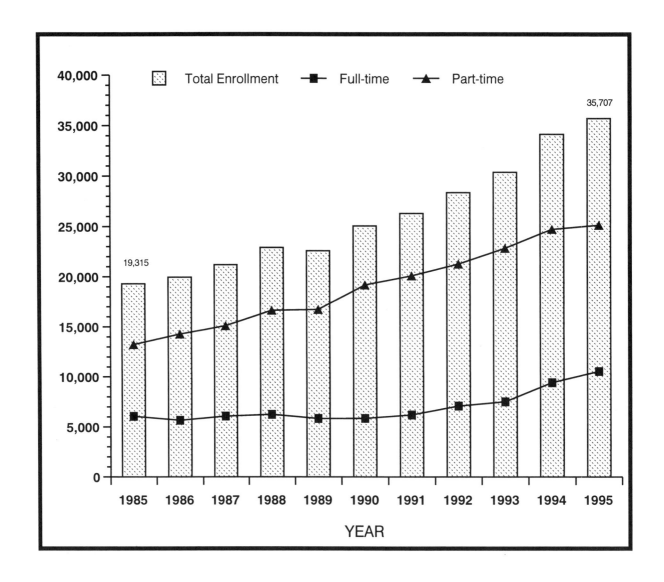

Figure 2. Master's Enrollments Increased To 35,707

In 1995, total enrollment in master's programs increased to 35,707, up 4.5 percent from the 1994 figure of 34,157. Full-time enrollment increased by 11.9 percent. Part-time enrollment increased by 1.7 percent and continued to account for an overwhelming 70.5 percent of the total enrollment.

Number Of Master's Graduates Continued To Rise

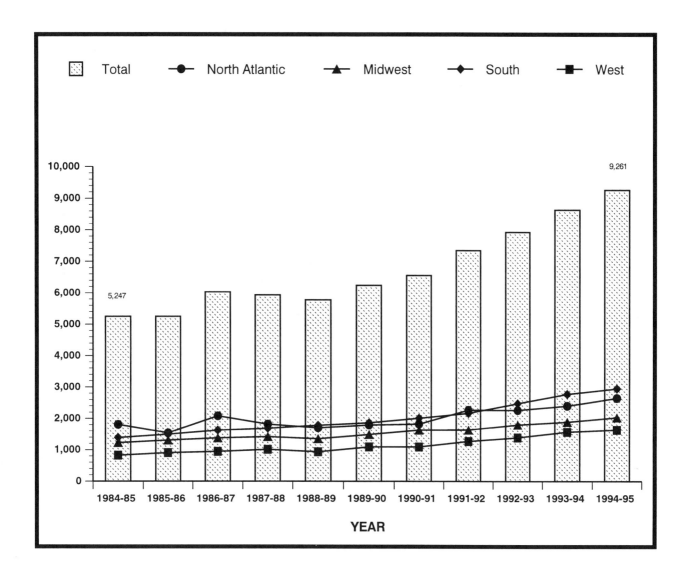

Figure 3.   Number Of Master's Graduates Continued To Rise

The number of graduates from master's programs increased by 7.3 percent, from 8,634 during the 1993-94 period to 9,261 in 1994-95. The South recorded the largest percentage of graduates at 31.8 percent and the West showed the smallest at 17.7 percent.

Number Of Doctoral Programs On An Upward Trend

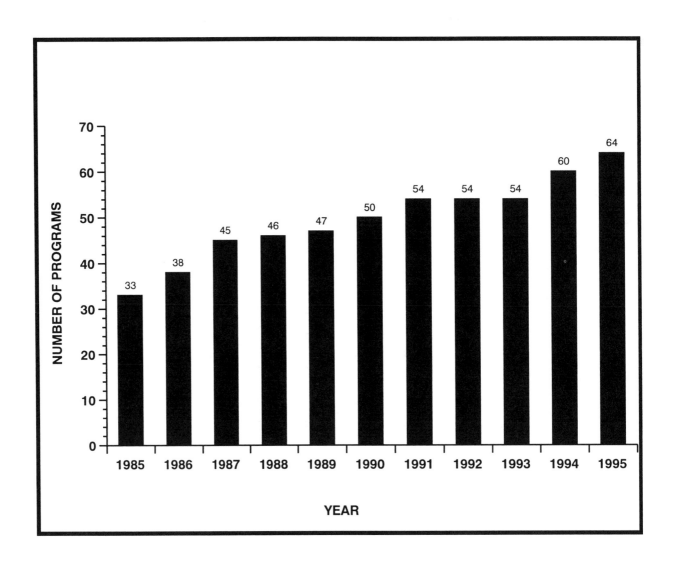

Figure 4. Number Of Doctoral Programs On An Upward Trend

The number of doctoral programs rose for the second consecutive year reaching a high of 64. The South had the greatest number of programs (20). The West had the fewest number of programs (8) and was the only region that had no new programs in 1995.

Doctoral Enrollments Still On The Rise

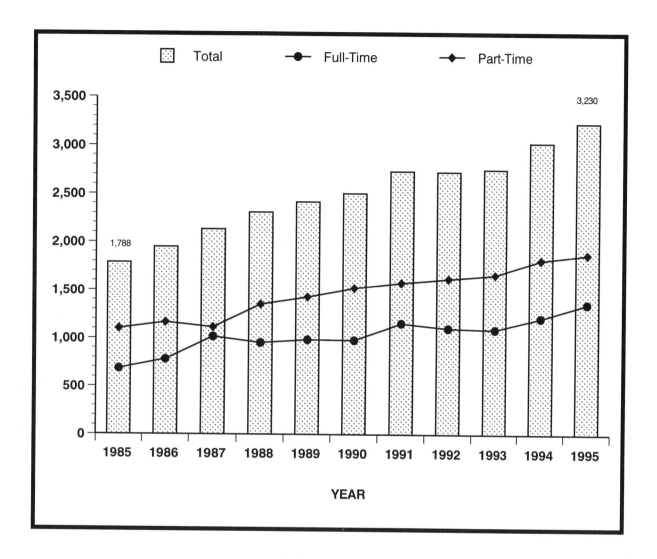

Figure 5. Doctoral Enrollments Still On The Rise

The number of students enrolled in doctoral programs rose to 3,230 in 1995, an increase of 6.7 percent. The highest number of enrollees were in programs located in the South (1,105) and the lowest were located in the West (427). The percentage of students enrolled part-time represented 58 percent of the total enrollment.

Doctoral Graduation Show An Increase After A Two Year Decline

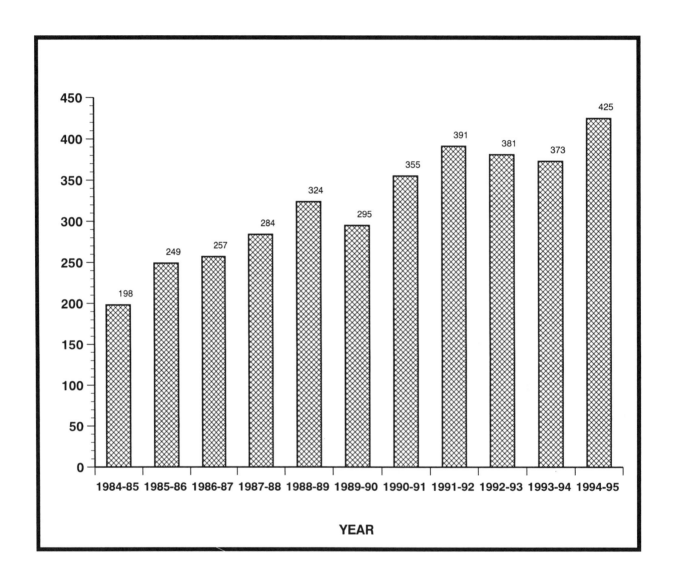

Figure 6.   Doctoral Graduations Show An Increase After A Two Year Decline

After a two year decline, graduation among doctoral students has shown an increase of 14 percent in the 1994-95 academic year. There were 425 graduates, most from programs in the South (144).

Master's Program Activities In International Education

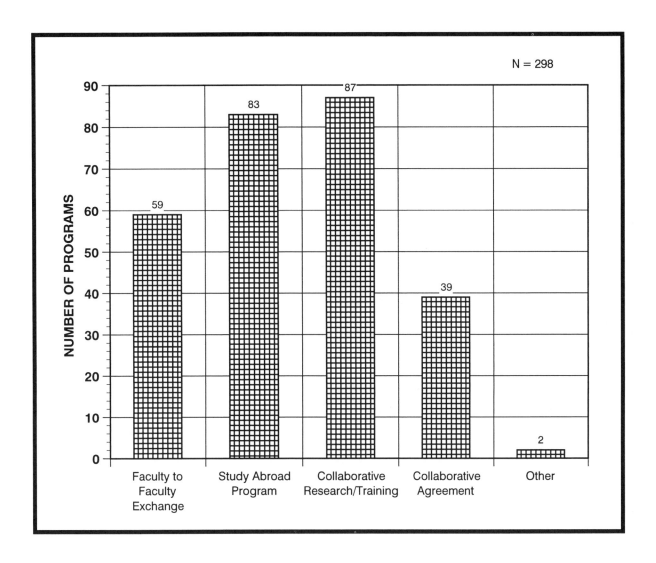

Figure 7   Master's Program Activities In International Education

A total of 87 (29.2 percent) master's programs reported that they were involved in collaborative research/teaching/training programs with international agencies or universities. Only 39 (13.1 percent) had collaborative agreements through non-governmental organizations (NGO).

Faculty Involved In Various Interdisciplinary Activities

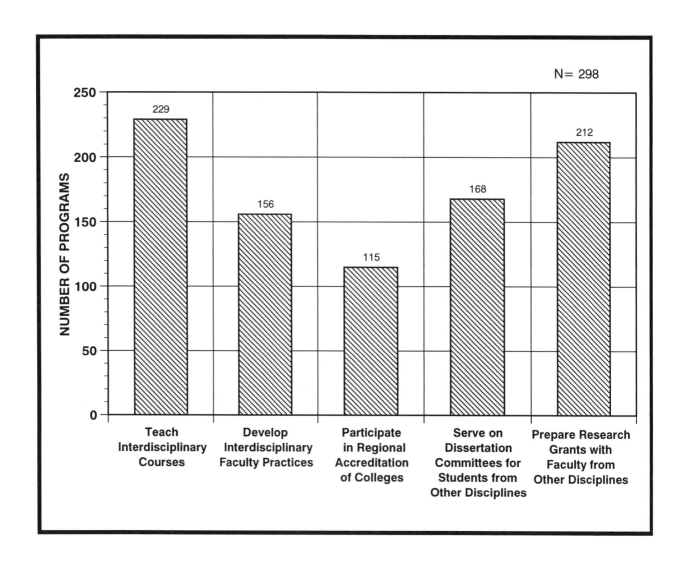

Figure 8.   Faculty Involved In Various Interdisciplinary Activities

Of the programs involved in interdisciplinary activities, over 70 percent of master's programs reported that members of their faculty were involved in the preparation of research grants with faculty from other disciplines. Seventy-seven percent taught interdisciplinary courses. Only 38.6 percent reported that their faculty participated in regional accreditation of colleges.

Nurse Practitioner Programs Remained The Most Common Speciality Among Master's Students

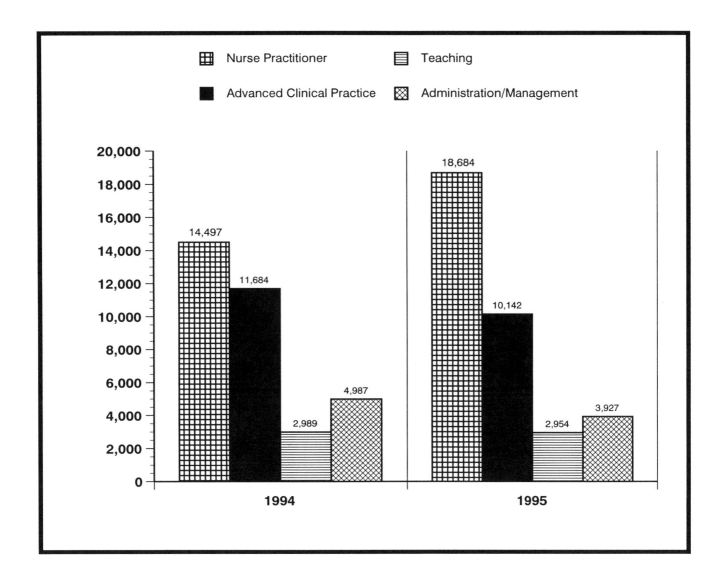

Figure 9. Nurse Practitioner Programs Remained The Most Common Specialty Among Master's Students

Nurse practitioner programs remain the specialty of choice for master's students for the second consecutive year. This is a change from 1993 when advanced clinical practice was the most common specialty. Teaching continues to be the specialty least often selected.

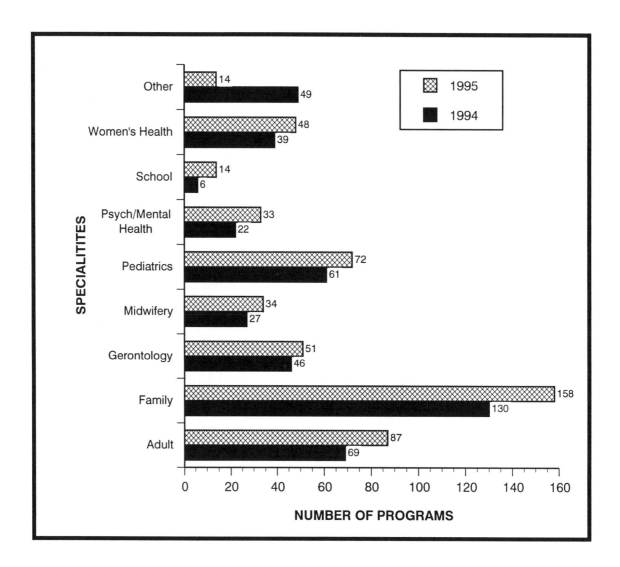

Figure 10. Nurse Practitioner Specialties Now Offered By 199 Master's Programs

A record high 199 (65 percent) master's programs offered nurse practitioner specialties. Family practice nursing remains the most popular area of study within nurse practitioner programs, followed by adult health.

Adult Health/Medical-Surgical Continues To Be The Most Popular Speciality In Advanced Clinical Practice

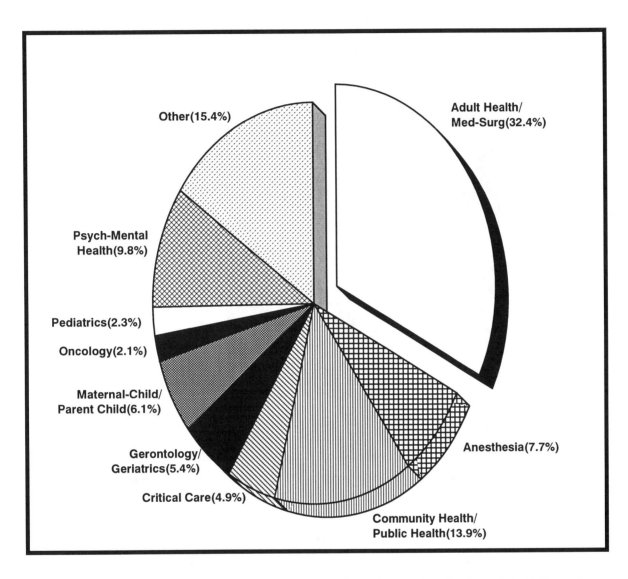

Figure 11. Adult Health/Medical-Surgical Continues To Be The Most Popular Specialty In Advanced Clinical Practice

A total of 10,142 students were enrolled in advanced clinical practice programs. Of this total, 32.4 percent concentrated their studies in adult health/medical surgical programs. Oncology recorded a minimum 2.1 percent of those enrolled.

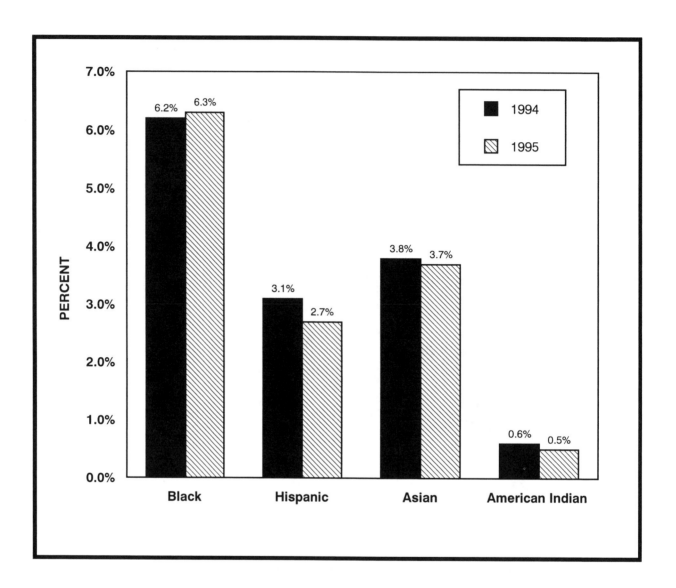

Figure 12. Enrollment Of Minority Students Show A Nominal Decline

The overall percentage of minority students enrolled has declined slightly (0.5 %) in 1995. Minority enrollment comprised 13.2 percent of total enrollments. Blacks, at 6.3 percent, represented the greatest sector of minorities and American Indians the smallest at 0.5 percent.

Graduation Of Minority Students Decreased By A Small Percent

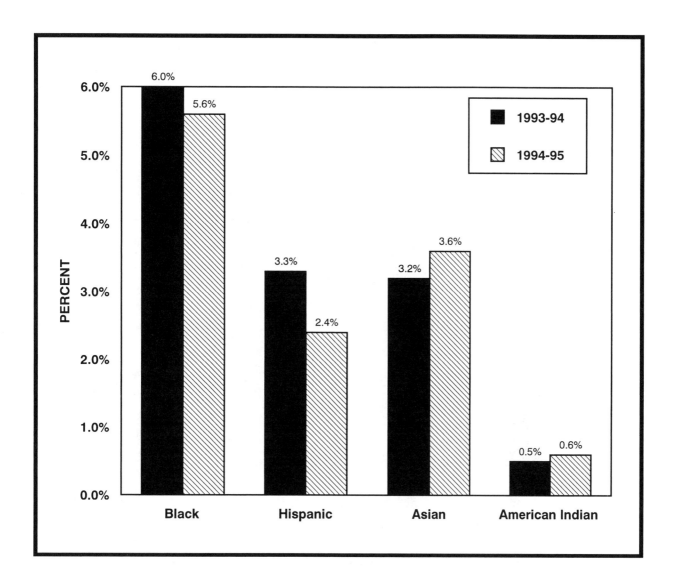

Figure 13. Graduation Of Minority Students Decreased By A Small Percent

The number of minorities graduating from master's programs has decreased slightly to 12.2 percent of the total number of graduates, down by 0.8 percent from 1994. The number of Asians and American Indians graduating increased but not enough to compensate for the decline in Hispanic graduates. The percentage of black graduates declined during 1994-95.

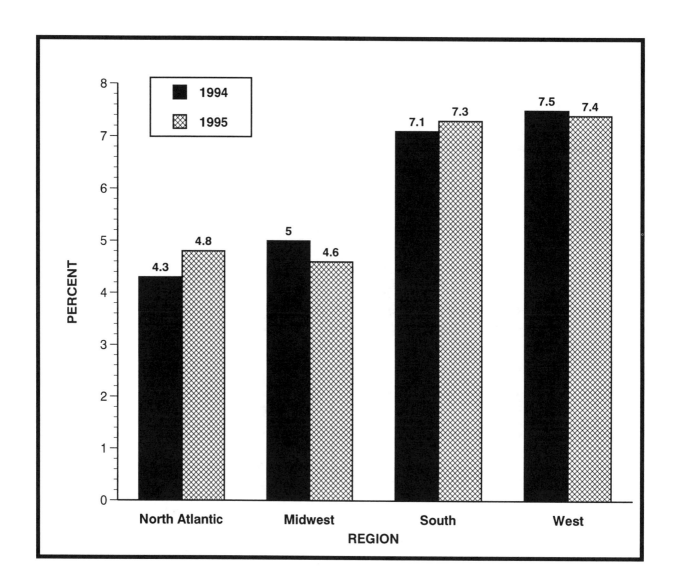

Figure 14. Largest Percentage Of Male Master's Students Were Found In The West

Males represented 5.9 percent of the total enrollment. The highest percentage (7.4 percent) of male students were found in the West, and the lowest were found in the Midwest region at 4.6 percent.

Section 2-3
Numeric Tables

Table 1
MASTER'S PROGRAMS IN NURSING, BY NLN REGION AND STATE: 1986 TO 1995[1]

NLN REGION AND STATE	NUMBER OF TOTAL PROGRAMS									
	1986	1987	1988	1989	1990	1991	1992	1993	1994	1995
United States	**189**	**194**	**197**	**212**	**231**	**236**	**243**	**252**	**276**	**306**
North Atlantic	48	52	53	57	67	68	71	76	82	90
Midwest	52	51	51	55	55	56	58	62	70	75
South	56	56	57	64	71	73	75	74	82	94
West	33	35	36	36	38	39	39	40	42	47
Alabama	4	4	4	4	4	4	4	4	5	6
Alaska	1	1	1	1	1	1	1	1	1	1
Arizona	2	2	2	2	2	2	2	2	2	4
Arkansas	2	2	2	2	2	3	3	3	3	3
California	16	17	17	17	18	18	18	19	19	19
Colorado	2	2	3	2	2	3	3	3	3	4
Connecticut	5	5	5	5	5	5	6	8	8	8
Delaware	1	1	1	1	1	1	1	2	2	2
District of Columbia	3	3	3	3	3	3	3	3	3	3
Florida	5	5	5	5	6	6	6	6	8	9
Georgia	4	4	4	6	7	7	7	7	7	10
Hawaii	1	1	1	1	1	1	1	1	1	1
Idaho	1	1	1	1	1	1	1	1	1	1
Illinois	10	10	10	10	12	11	11	12	12	13
Indiana	6	6	6	7	7	7	7	7	9	9
Iowa	2	2	2	2	2	2	2	2	2	2
Kansas	2	2	2	2	3	3	3	4	4	4
Kentucky	4	4	4	5	5	5	5	5	6	8
Louisiana	2	2	2	3	4	3	4	4	4	5
Maine	1	1	1	1	1	1	2	2	3	3
Maryland	2	2	3	3	3	3	3	3	4	4
Massachusetts	6	7	6	6	10	10	10	11	11	11
Michigan	9	8	8	10	9	9	9	10	10	10
Minnesota	3	3	3	4	3	3	4	4	5	6
Mississippi	3	3	3	3	3	3	3	3	3	5
Missouri	3	3	3	3	3	3	3	4	6	7
Montana	1	1	1	1	1	1	1	1	1	1
Nebraska	2	2	2	2	2	3	3	3	3	3
Nevada	2	2	2	2	2	2	2	2	2	2
New Hampshire	1	1	1	1	1	1	1	1	2	2
New Jersey	2	2	2	2	3	3	3	3	5	8
New Mexico	1	1	1	1	1	1	1	1	1	2
New York	17	18	19	20	23	23	23	24	25	26
North Carolina	6	6	6	7	7	7	7	6	6	6
North Dakota	2	2	2	2	2	2	2	2	2	2
Ohio	7	7	7	7	6	7	8	8	10	10
Oklahoma	2	2	2	3	2	2	3	3	2	2
Oregon	2	2	2	2	2	2	2	2	2	2
Pennsylvania	11	13	14	16	18	19	20	20	21	25
Rhode Island	1	1	1	1	1	1	1	1	1	1
South Carolina	3	3	3	3	3	3	3	3	3	3
South Dakota	1	1	1	1	1	1	1	1	1	2
Tennessee	3	3	3	2	3	5	5	5	6	7
Texas	9	9	9	10	13	13	13	13	15	15
Utah	2	2	2	2	2	2	2	2	2	3
Vermont	0	0	0	1	1	1	1	1	1	1
Virginia	6	6	6	6	7	7	7	7	7	8
Washington	2	2	2	3	4	4	4	4	6	6
West Virginia	1	1	1	2	2	2	2	2	3	3
Wisconsin	5	5	5	5	5	5	5	5	6	7
Wyoming	1	1	1	1	1	1	1	1	1	1
American Samoa	0	0	0	0	0	0	0	0	0	0
Guam	0	0	0	1	0	0	0	0	0	0
Puerto Rico	1	2	2	2	2	2	2	2	2	2
Virgin Islands	0	0	0	0	0	0	0	0	0	0

[1]National and regional totals exclude American Samoa, Guam, Puerto Rico, and the Virgin Islands.

Table 2
NURSE PRACTITIONER PROGRAMS IN MASTER'S PROGRAMS,
BY AREA OF SPECIALIZATION AND NLN REGION: 1994-1995[1,2]

	UNITED STATES	NORTH ATLANTIC	MIDWEST	SOUTH	WEST
Total	**199**	**60**	**42**	**67**	**30**
Adult	87	27	19	28	13
Family	158	42	32	59	25
Gerontology	51	13	15	17	6
Midwifery	34	8	7	10	9
Pediatrics	72	21	16	24	11
Psych-Mental Health	33	9	4	13	7
School	14	3	2	2	7
Women's Health	48	12	11	18	7
Other	14	3	5	4	2

[1]Excludes American Samoa, Guam, Puerto Rico, and the Virgin Islands.
[2]Master's programs can offer more than one type of nurse practitioner program.

Table 3
ENROLLMENTS OF NURSES IN MASTER'S PROGRAMS AND PERCENTAGE
IN NLN-ACCREDITED PROGRAMS: 1975 TO 1995[1]

PROGRAMS ACADEMIC YEAR			ENROLLMENTS					
			Total		Full-Time		Part-Time	
	Number	Percent Accredited	Number	Percent Accredited	Number	Percent Accredited	Number	Percent Accredited
1975	99	69.0	9,662	90.6	5,402	93.4	4,260	87.1
1976	103	67.9	10,809	88.4	5,924	92.5	4,885	83.4
1977	112*	66.4	12,143	86.8	6,112	92.5	6,031	81.0
1978	117	68.1	13,105	87.0	6,561	91.5	6,544	82.5
1979	125	72.4	14,130	87.8	6,891	91.8	7,239	83.9
1980	135	66.4	15,053	86.3	7,306	89.0	7,747	83.7
1981	140	65.5	16,125	85.2	7,000	87.3	9,125	83.6
1982	151	78.1	17,085	91.1	6,389	96.0	10,696	88.2
1983	154	77.5	18,112	87.6	6,478	89.8	11,634	86.3
1984	166	82.7	18,822	95.1	6,587	93.0	12,235	97.3
1985	167	83.1	19,315	93.3	6,057	98.1	13,258	91.2
1986	189	74.6	19,958	87.3	5,664	94.6	14,294	82.3
1987	194	91.6	21,195	90.8	6,113	93.5	15,082	89.4
1988	197	78.2	22,908	91.4	6,253	95.5	16,655	89.8
1989	212	80.7	22,587	92.2	5,860	94.9	16,727	91.2
1990	231	78.4	25,065[†]	90.6[†]	5,887[†]	90.2	19,178[†]	90.7[†]
1991	236	82.6	26,308	93.0	6,212	95.0	20,096	92.4
1992	243	84.4	28,370	93.9	7,083	95.4	21,287	93.5
1993	252	88.9	30,385	96.3	7,539	96.6	22,846	96.3
1994	276	83.3	34,157	94.0	9,427	94.6	24,730	93.8
1995	306	75.2	35,707	91.1	10,553	88.5	25,154	92.2

[†] Excludes American Samoa, Guam, Puerto Rico, and the Virgin Islands.
* One school shown in the total number of programs reported no enrollments for 1977.
[†] Due to an error in 1990 enrollments, totals and percentages have been changed for that year.

Table 4
ENROLLMENTS OF NURSES IN MASTER'S PROGRAMS,
PERCENTAGE CHANGE FROM PREVIOUS YEAR, AND PERCENTAGE ENROLLED FULL-TIME,
BY NLN REGION: 1975 TO 1995[1]

YEAR	ALL REGIONS				NORTH ATLANTIC				MIDWESTERN				SOUTHERN				WESTERN			
	Number of Programs	Enrollments			Number of Programs	Enrollments			Number of Programs	Enrollments			Number of Programs	Enrollments			Number of Programs	Enrollments		
		Number	Percent Change	Percent Full Time		Number	Percent Change	Percent Full Time		Number	Percent Change	Percent Full Time		Number	Percent Change	Percent Full Time		Number	Percent Change	Percent Full Time
1975	100	9,662	+21.9	55.9	24	3,337	+24.1	51.5	28	2,252	+14.8	54.6	29	2,358	+28.6	52.3	19	1,715	+19.1	71.7
1976	106	10,809	+11.9	54.8	26	3,853	+15.5	50.8	28	2,409	+7.0	55.0	33	2,805	+19.0	51.1	19	1,742	+1.6	69.3
1977	114	12,143	+12.3	50.3	26	3,994	+3.7	50.4	31*	3,001	+24.6	47.2	40	3,281	+17.0	43.6	17	1,867	+7.2	67.3
1978	119	13,105	+7.9	50.1	29	4,344	+8.8	48.9	31	3,129	+4.3	45.1	40	3,454	+5.3	46.0	19	2,178	+16.7	65.8
1979	127	14,130	+7.8	48.8	29	4,068	-6.4	48.5	32	3,796	+21.3	44.6	46	3,942	+14.1	42.5	20	2,324	+6.7	66.7
1980	137	15,053	+6.5	48.5	32	4,472	+9.9	51.1	34	4,146	+9.2	40.6	48	3,964	+0.6	43.6	23	2,471	+6.3	65.0
1981	142	16,125	+7.1	43.4	34	4,848	+8.4	43.8	37	4,254	+2.6	35.9	48	4,390	+10.7	41.3	23	2,633	+6.6	58.4
1982	151	17,085	+6.3	37.4	37	5,344	+10.2	33.2	40	4,467	+5.0	29.0	52	4,561	+5.2	38.2	24	2,713	+3.0	57.7
1983	154	18,112	+6.5	34.6	37	5,830	+9.1	30.0	40	4,680	+4.8	27.2	51	4,807	+7.3	36.0	26	2,593	-4.4	59.1
1984	166	18,822	+3.9	35.0	42	5,861	+0.5	26.9	44	4,780	+2.1	35.5	54	5,403	+12.4	29.7	26	2,778	+7.1	61.6
1985	167	19,315	+2.6	31.4	42	5,837	-0.4	23.4	44	5,327	+11.4	24.6	54	5,330	-1.4	34.0	27	2,821	+1.5	44.2
1986	189	19,958	+3.3	28.4	48	5,883	+0.7	21.9	52	5,400	+1.4	20.1	56	5,590	+4.9	32.4	33	3,085	+9.4	47.9
1987	194	21,195	+6.2	28.7	52	6,380	+8.4	20.7	51	5,505	+1.9	21.5	56	6,004	+7.4	33.7	35	3,306	+7.1	47.5
1988	197	22,908	+8.1	27.3	53	7,425	+16.4	18.7	51	5,720	+3.9	19.1	57	5,986	-0.3	30.7	36	3,777	+14.3	50.9
1989	212	22,587	-1.4	25.9	57	6,313	-15.0	18.8	55	5,970	+4.4	16.9	64	6,581	+9.9	29.5	36	3,723	-1.4	46.1
1990	231	25,065'	+11.0'	23.4'	67	7,105	+12.5	17.2	55	6,128	+2.6	17.1	71	7,540'	+14.6'	28.4'	38	4,292	+15.3	34.4
1991	236	26,308	+5.0	23.6	73	7,520	+5.8	17.2	56	6,258	+2.1	15.9	73	8,067	+7.0	25.7	39	4,463	+4.0	41.3
1992	243	28,370	+7.8	25.0	71	8,280	+10.1	19.2	58	6,833	+9.2	15.5	75	8,650	+7.2	27.5	39	4,607	+3.2	44.5
1993	252	30,385	+7.1	24.8	76	8,988	+8.6	16.8	62	7,401	+8.3	18.2	74	8,956	+3.5	28.2	40	5,040	+9.4	42.6
1994	276	34,157	+12.4	27.6	82	9,930	+10.5	19.7	70	8,711	+17.7	17.9	82	10,437	+16.5	34.4	42	5,079	+0.8	27.9
1995	306	35,707	+4.5	29.6	90	10,654	+7.3	20.0	75	9,155	+5.1	20.4	94	10,386	-0.5	32.8	47	5,512	+8.5	57.1

[1] Excludes American Samoa, Guam, Puerto Rico, and the Virgin Islands.

* One school shown in the total number of programs reported no enrollments for 1977.

' Due to an error in 1990 enrollments in West Virginia, the total and southern region numbers and percentages have been changed for that year.

Table 5
ENROLLMENTS OF REGISTERED NURSES IN MASTER'S PROGRAMS IN NURSING, BY NLN REGION AND STATE: 1986 TO 1995[1]

NLN REGION AND STATE	NUMBER OF ENROLLMENTS IN MASTER'S PROGRAMS									
	1986	1987	1988	1989	1990	1991	1992	1993	1994	1995
United States	**19,958**	**21,195**	**22,908**	**22,587**	**25,065***	**26,308**	**28,370**	**30,385**	**34,157**	**35,707**
North Atlantic	5,883	6,380	7,425	6,313	7,105	7,520	8,280	8,988	9,930	10,654
Midwest	5,400	5,505	5,720	5,970	6,128	6,258	6,833	7,401	8,711	9,155
South	5,590	6,004	5,986	6,581	7,540*	8,067	8,650	8,956	10,437	10,386
West	3,085	3,306	3,777	3,723	4,292	4,463	4,607	5,040	5,079	5,512
Alabama	369	446	413	446	493	430	455	493	626	805
Alaska	18	18	18	33	44	44	46	47	49	40
Arizona	246	263	308	322	336	297	280	316	343	773
Arkansas	154	159	144	128	159	198	214	250	312	325
California	1,640	1,692	1,913	1,905	2,456	2,565	2,616	2,922	2,696	2,554
Colorado	200	262	431	240	234	300	329	317	321	480
Connecticut	439	472	501	481	489	467	530	645	716	712
Delaware	87	73	82	77	86	64	76	143	216	185
District of Columbia	328	305	268	275	301	309	261	270	317	291
Florida	497	513	576	674	881	938	1,049	1,031	1,270	1,397
Georgia	404	428	455	490	581	604	659	742	841	862
Hawaii	55	52	60	65	67	99	110	106	115	117
Idaho	49	41	41	80	57	63	50	76	71	22
Illinois	936	1,005	953	979	1,014	911	1,013	1,167	1,376	1,476
Indiana	519	703	663	681	692	554	585	799	947	994
Iowa	209	285	294	250	309	289	292	297	300	288
Kansas	287	265	285	287	320	367	422	515	528	531
Kentucky	180	147	189	512	437	425	427	448	648	448
Louisiana	235	220	202	230	256	282	338	354	421	321
Maine	78	50	44	57	74	91	112	117	138	131
Maryland	398	394	437	526	530	666	686	666	720	792
Massachusetts	489	657	558	516	766	732	1,062	1,189	1,409	1,530
Michigan	957	748	802	961	958	990	1,112	1,133	1,239	1,396
Minnesota	172	164	167	207	217	242	363	387	442	476
Mississippi	115	128	147	152	139	184	205	271	247	245
Missouri	426	452	457	473	519	545	589	558	981	873
Montana	22	24	20	23	23	31	31	33	37	41
Nebraska	120	77	156	172	191	272	276	226	255	336
Nevada	34	65	55	94	83	71	66	59	37	83
New Hampshire	35	54	41	36	32	35	40	62	207	187
New Jersey	276	345	251	264	321	353	357	415	404	748
New Mexico	35	59	81	92	117	119	130	113	142	158
New York	2,803	2,827	4,023	2,968	3,290	3,566	3,704	3,909	4,303	4,450
North Carolina	412	501	511	510	618	639	790	787	948	932
North Dakota	101	92	104	116	132	134	122	131	177	175
Ohio	1,064	1,113	1,204	1,218	1,133	1,264	1,360	1,415	1,590	1,672
Oklahoma	162	163	163	176	141	143	181	224	245	268
Oregon	173	224	227	276	252	207	230	232	233	232
Pennsylvania	1,260	1,507	1,535	1,539	1,620	1,784	2,023	2,114	2,094	2,264
Rhode Island	88	90	122	89	94	77	79	88	97	112
South Carolina	308	368	384	440	444	404	405	399	442	388
South Dakota	76	58	115	114	134	163	128	171	153	180
Tennessee	308	379	349	204	397	530	649	741	674	634
Texas	1,356	1,389	1,378	1,450	1,696	1,769	1,795	1,728	2,054	1,952
Utah	257	238	234	217	221	201	228	283	278	293
Vermont	0	0	0	11	32	42	36	36	29	44
Virginia	582	699	585	524	679	724	638	656	803	807
Washington	304	312	334	320	341	404	426	471	693	656
West Virginia	110	70	53	119	89*	131	159	166	186	210
Wisconsin	533	543	520	512	509	527	571	602	723	758
Wyoming	52	56	55	56	61	62	65	65	64	63
American Samoa	0	0	0	0	0	0	0	0	0	0
Guam	0	0	0	51	0	0	0	0	0	0
Puerto Rico	95	155	160	161	126	160	146	200	187	209
Virgin Islands	0	0	0	0	0	0	0	0	0	0

[1] National and regional totals exclude American Samoa, Guam, Puerto Rico, and the Virgin Islands.

* Due to an error in 1990 enrollments in West Virginia, the total, south, and West Virginia numbers have been changed for that year.

Table 6
FULL-TIME ENROLLMENTS OF NURSES IN MASTER'S PROGRAMS, BY FUNCTIONAL AREA OF STUDY: 1993-1995[1]

YEAR	TOTAL		NURSE PRACTITIONERS		ADVANCED CLINICAL PRACTICE		TEACHING		ADMINISTRATION/ MANAGEMENT		OTHER	
	Number	Percent	Number	Percent	Number	Percent	Number	Percent	Number	Percent	Number	Percent
1993	7,539	100.0	2,876	38.1	2,969	39.4	519	6.9	781	10.4	394	5.2
1994	9,427	100.0	5,317	56.4	3,098	32.9	371	3.9	641	6.8	0	0.0
1995	10,553	100.0	6,654	63.0	2,658	25.2	576	5.5	665	6.3	0	0.0

[1] Excludes American Samoa, Guam, Puerto Rico, and the Virgin Islands.

Table 6A
FULL-TIME ENROLLMENTS IN NURSE PRACTITIONER PROGRAMS, BY NURSING CONTENT AREA: 1993-1995[1]

	1993		1994		1995	
	Number	Percent	Number	Percent	Number	Percent
Total	**2,876**	**100.0**	**5,317**	**100.0**	**6,654**	**100.0**
Adult	309	10.7	814	15.3	1,041	15.6
Family	1,382	48.1	2,559	48.1	3,280	49.3
Gerontology	147	5.1	203	3.8	264	4.0
Midwifery	281	9.8	333	6.3	439	6.6
Pediatric	325	11.3	637	12.0	616	9.3
Psych/Mental Health	73	2.5	112	2.1	135	2.0
School	13	0.5	3	0.1	35	0.5
Women's Health	183	6.4	272	5.1	322	4.8
Other	163	5.7	384	7.2	522	7.8

[1] Excludes American Samoa, Guam, Puerto Rico, and the Virgin Islands.

Table 6B
FULL-TIME ENROLLMENTS OF NURSES IN ADVANCED CLINICAL PRACTICE, BY NURSING CONTENT AREA: 1993-1995[1]

	1993		1994		1995	
	Number	Percent	Number	Percent	Number	Percent
Total	**2,969**	**100.0**	**3,098**	**100.0**	**2,658**	**100.0**
Adult Health/Med-Surg	603	20.3	658	21.2	589	22.2
Anesthesia	399	13.4	699	22.6	619	23.3
Community Health/ Public Health	358	12.1	395	12.8	369	13.9
Critical Care	267	9.0	262	8.5	108	4.1
Gerontology/Geriatrics	86	2.9	80	2.6	104	3.9
Maternal-Child/ Parent-Child	324	10.9	217	7.0	129	4.8
Oncology	64	2.2	57	1.8	49	1.8
Pediatric	98	3.3	78	2.5	58	2.2
Psych-Mental Health	310	10.4	319	10.3	258	9.7
Other	460	15.5	333	10.7	375	14.1

[1] Excludes American Samoa, Guam, Puerto Rico, and the Virgin Islands.

Table 6C
FULL-TIME ENROLLMENTS OF NURSES
IN TEACHING, BY NURSING CONTENT AREA: 1993-1995[1]

	1993		1994		1995	
	Number	Percent	Number	Percent	Number	Percent
Total	**519**	**100.0**	**371**	**100.0**	**576**	**100.0**
Adult Health/Med-Surg	201	38.7	118	31.8	102	17.7
Anesthesia	8	1.5	3	0.8	1	0.2
Community Health/ Public Health	36	6.9	29	7.8	28	4.9
Critical Care	16	3.1	5	1.3	10	1.7
Gerontology/Geriatrics	25	4.8	16	4.3	11	1.9
Maternal-Child/ Parent-Child	36	6.9	22	5.9	5	0.9
Oncology	2	0.4	0	0.0	10	1.7
Pediatric	11	2.1	7	1.9	16	2.8
Psych-Mental Health	48	9.2	8	2.2	7	1.2
Other	136	26.2	163	44.0	386	67.0

[1] Excludes American Samoa, Guam, Puerto Rico, and the Virgin Islands.

Table 7
PART-TIME ENROLLMENTS OF NURSES IN MASTER'S PROGRAMS,
BY FUNCTIONAL AREA OF STUDY: 1993-1995[1]

YEAR	TOTAL		NURSE PRACTITIONERS		ADVANCED CLINICAL PRACTICE		TEACHING		ADMINISTRATION/ MANAGEMENT		OTHER	
	Number	Percent	Number	Percent	Number	Percent	Number	Percent	Number	Percent	Number	Percent
1993	22,846	100.0	5,220	22.8	8,250	36.1	2,507	11.0	5,110	22.4	1,759	7.7
1994	24,730	100.0	9,180	37.1	8,586	34.7	2,618	10.6	4,346	17.6	0	0.0
1995	25,154	100.0	12,030	47.8	7,484	29.8	2,378	9.5	3,262	12.9	0	0.0

[1] Excludes American Samoa, Guam, Puerto Rico, and the Virgin Islands.

Table 7A
PART-TIME ENROLLMENTS IN NURSE PRACTITIONER
PROGRAMS, BY NURSING CONTENT AREA: 1993-1995[1]

	1993		1994		1995	
	Number	Percent	Number	Percent	Number	Percent
Total	**5,220**	**100.0**	**9,180**	**100.0**	**12,030**	**100.0**
Adult	1,128	21.6	2,252	24.5	2,918	24.3
Family	2,053	39.3	3,548	38.6	4,713	39.2
Gerontology	268	5.1	428	4.7	436	3.6
Midwifery	157	3.0	297	3.2	302	2.5
Pediatric	720	13.8	1,074	11.7	1,255	10.4
Psych/Mental Health	123	2.4	252	2.7	312	2.6
School	23	0.4	29	0.3	49	0.4
Women's Health	266	5.1	417	4.5	495	4.1
Other	482	9.2	883	9.6	1,550	12.9

[1] Excludes American Samoa, Guam, Puerto Rico, and the Virgin Islands.

Table 7B
PART-TIME ENROLLMENTS OF NURSES IN ADVANCED CLINICAL PRACTICE, BY NURSING CONTENT AREA: 1993-1995[1]

	1993		1994		1995	
	Number	Percent	Number	Percent	Number	Percent
Total	**8,250**	**100.0**	**8,586**	**100.0**	**7,484**	**100.0**
Adult Health/Med-Surg	2,781	33.7	3,124	36.4	2,693	35.9
Anesthesia	162	2.0	117	1.4	159	2.1
Community Health/ Public Health	898	10.9	1,067	12.4	1,038	13.8
Critical Care	726	8.8	610	7.1	392	5.2
Gerontology/Geriatrics	347	4.2	408	4.8	446	5.9
Maternal-Child/ Parent-Child	813	9.9	664	7.7	487	6.5
Oncology	198	2.4	201	2.3	162	2.2
Pediatric	342	4.1	331	3.9	176	2.4
Psych-Mental Health	914	11.1	919	10.7	740	10.0
Other	1,069	13.0	1,145	13.3	1,191	16.0

[1] Excludes American Samoa, Guam, Puerto Rico, and the Virgin Islands.

Table 7C
PART-TIME ENROLLMENTS OF NURSES IN TEACHING, BY NURSING CONTENT AREA: 1993-1995[1]

	1993		1994		1995	
	Number	Percent	Number	Percent	Number	Percent
Total	**2,507**	**100.0**	**2,618**	**100.0**	**2,378**	**100.0**
Adult Health/Med-Surg	985	39.3	903	34.6	862	36.2
Anesthesia	0	0.0	11	0.4	28	1.1
Community Health/ Public Health	179	7.1	184	7.0	164	6.9
Critical Care	57	2.3	45	1.7	40	1.7
Gerontology/Geriatrics	86	3.4	66	2.5	149	6.3
Maternal-Child/ Parent-Child	125	5.0	110	4.2	33	1.4
Oncology	28	1.1	10	0.4	58	2.4
Pediatric	66	2.6	66	2.5	75	3.2
Psych-Mental Health	73	2.9	64	2.4	71	3.0
Other	908	36.2	1,159	44.3	898	37.8

[1] Excludes American Samoa, Guam, Puerto Rico, and the Virgin Islands.

Table 8
GRADUATIONS FROM MASTER'S PROGRAMS AND PERCENTAGE CHANGE FROM PREVIOUS YEAR, BY NLN REGION: 1974-75 TO 1994-95[1]

ACADEMIC YEAR	ALL REGIONS			NORTH ATLANTIC			MIDWESTERN			SOUTHERN			WESTERN		
	Number of Programs	Number	Percent Change	Number of Programs	Number	Percent Change	Number of Programs	Number	Percent Change	Number of Programs	Number	Percent Change	Number of Programs	Number	Percent Change
1974-75	100	2,678	+2.1	24	955	+4.8	28	516	-4.3	29	642	+6.5	19	565	-1.0
1975-76	106	3,417	+27.6	26	1,186	+24.2	28	688	+33.3	33	854	+33.0	19	689	+21.9
1976-77	102	3,800	+11.2	24	1,284	+8.3	28	857	+24.6	33	1,027	+20.6	17	632	-8.3
1977-78	109	4,255	+12.0	26	1,573	+22.5	24	915	+6.8	37	1,145	+11.5	17	622	-1.6
1978-79	118	4,596	+8.0	27	1,630	+3.6	32	986	+7.8	41	1,307	+14.1	18	673	+8.2
1979-80	121	4,755	+3.5	29	1,565	-4.0	32	1,068	+8.3	41	1,333	+2.0	19	789	+17.2
1980-81	127	4,998	+5.1	30	1,472	-5.9	30	1,207	+13.0	46	1,510	+13.3	21	809	+2.5
1981-82	138	5,149	+3.0	32	1,530	+3.9	34	1,289	+6.8	48	1,463	-3.1	24	867	+7.1
1982-83	141	5,039	-2.1	34	1,565	+2.3	38	1,230	-4.6	45	1,325	-12.1	24	919	+6.0
1983-84	164*	5,082	+0.9	42	1,641	+4.7	44	1,165	-5.6	52	1,388	+4.6	26	888	-3.5
1984-85	167	5,247	+3.2	42	1,808	+10.2	44	1,224	+5.1	54	1,389	+0.1	27	826	-7.0
1985-86	189	5,248	-0.0	48	1,541	-14.8	52	1,306	+6.7	56	1,496	+7.7	33	905	+9.6
1986-87	194	6,029	+14.9	52	2,080	+35.0	51	1,376	+5.3	56	1,628	+8.8	35	945	+4.4
1987-88	197	5,933	-1.6	53	1,817	-12.6	51	1,419	+3.1	57	1,686	+3.6	36	1,011	+7.0
1988-89	212	5,777	-2.6	57	1,703	-6.3	55	1,354	-4.6	64	1,782	+5.7	36	938	-7.2
1989-90	231	6,243	+8.1	67	1,791	+5.2	55	1,491	+10.1	71	1,865	+4.6	38	1,096	+16.8
1990-91	236	6,555	+5.0	68	1,822	+1.7	56	1,629	+9.2	73	2,011	+7.8	39	1,093	-0.3
1991-92	243	7,345	+12.1	71	2,271	+24.6	58	1,636	+0.4	75	2,168	+7.8	39	1,270	+16.2
1992-93	252	7,926	+7.9	76	2,264	-0.3	62	1,800	+10.0	74	2,476	+14.2	40	1,386	+9.1
1993-94	276	8,634	+8.9	82	2,401	+6.1	70	1,888	+4.8	82	2,775	+12.1	42	1,570	+13.3
1994-95	306	9,261	+7.3	90	2,650	+10.4	75	2,030	+7.5	94	2,946	+6.2	47	1,635	+4.1

[1] Excludes American Samoa, Guam, Puerto Rico, and the Virgin Islands.
* Two programs had not yet graduated their first class at time of reporting.
[†] A previously unreported program was included.

Table 9
GRADUATIONS OF REGISTERED NURSES FROM MASTER'S PROGRAMS IN NURSING,
BY NLN REGION AND STATE: 1985-86 TO 1994-95[1]

NLN REGION AND STATE	NUMBER OF GRADUATIONS FROM MASTER'S PROGRAMS									
	1985-86	1986-87	1987-88	1988-89	1989-90	1990-91	1991-92	1992-93	1993-94	1994-95
United States	**5,248**	**6,029**	**5,933**	**5,777**	**6,243**	**6,555**	**7,345**	**7,926**	**8,634**	**9,261**
North Atlantic	1,541	2,080	1,817	1,703	1,791	1,822	2,271	2,264	2,401	2,650
Midwest	1,306	1,376	1,419	1,354	1,491	1,629	1,636	1,800	1,888	2,030
South	1,496	1,628	1,686	1,782	1,865	2,011	2,168	2,476	2,775	2,946
West	905	945	1,011	938	1,096	1,093	1,270	1,386	1,570	1,635
Alabama	150	132	146	134	147	208	189	166	186	224
Alaska	12	0	0	2	8	1	13	17	11	10
Arizona	65	55	56	48	72	74	89	79	126	230
Arkansas	18	21	30	42	25	32	42	57	58	65
California	477	517	436	500	570	581	637	732	892	755
Colorado	70	80	218	83	85	73	78	141	121	139
Connecticut	93	117	115	110	126	130	130	154	182	151
Delaware	26	27	19	22	18	19	27	19	12	53
District of Columbia	131	116	131	100	78	72	114	76	127	109
Florida	96	151	124	129	193	184	191	236	297	321
Georgia	123	97	122	122	148	173	146	203	190	232
Hawaii	9	23	20	7	30	16	39	32	38	36
Idaho	7	2	8	10	7	7	11	11	13	27
Illinois	294	328	261	294	406	413	353	341	355	375
Indiana	172	165	157	160	151	117	221	157	149	182
Iowa	25	17	18	26	24	62	68	51	73	50
Kansas	72	76	69	65	67	72	66	89	121	127
Kentucky	70	47	43	139	84	133	89	80	91	71
Louisiana	86	65	51	48	60	37	35	58	61	113
Maine	7	17	17	13	14	17	20	32	34	19
Maryland	99	113	109	106	114	127	176	181	174	205
Massachusetts	144	480	175	165	302	231	327	347	322	433
Michigan	184	170	179	152	167	207	184	253	232	234
Minnesota	68	103	126	68	100	67	67	101	99	133
Mississippi	37	43	43	59	75	53	61	96	85	112
Missouri	76	83	82	112	104	91	136	155	162	177
Montana	7	3	9	5	4	9	0	6	9	5
Nebraska	31	17	29	26	22	33	36	60	53	50
Nevada	7	8	5	7	10	9	19	27	7	10
New Hampshire	0	2	4	6	10	6	6	5	9	27
New Jersey	79	99	88	64	50	54	54	96	108	110
New Mexico	21	14	16	12	18	34	45	43	40	37
New York	645	645	772	680	731	742	953	911	949	1,113
North Carolina	103	87	112	129	134	129	158	176	257	235
North Dakota	6	26	18	22	25	40	42	28	38	49
Ohio	242	260	356	284	277	390	323	408	406	459
Oklahoma	54	57	42	43	47	41	47	40	55	49
Oregon	56	49	65	77	86	107	129	85	94	121
Pennsylvania	403	558	468	523	435	521	596	576	607	607
Rhode Island	13	19	28	20	27	27	27	30	29	26
South Carolina	50	61	89	110	119	131	144	129	158	116
South Dakota	14	15	6	10	16	11	19	32	47	24
Tennessee	84	109	113	54	158	156	169	224	275	330
Texas	320	352	380	413	361	330	439	515	578	564
Utah	47	54	61	65	60	46	66	57	66	82
Vermont	0	0	0	0	0	3	17	18	22	2
Virginia	174	261	244	229	184	259	261	277	264	269
Washington	123	134	109	105	133	131	130	145	139	171
West Virginia	32	32	38	25	16	18	21	38	46	40
Wisconsin	122	116	118	135	132	126	121	125	153	170
Wyoming	4	6	8	17	13	5	14	11	14	12
American Samoa	0	0	0	0	0	0	0	0	0	0
Guam	0	0	0	23	0	0	0	0	0	0
Puerto Rico	59	65	45	57	40	0	42	40	88	62
Virgin Islands	0	0	0	0	0	0	0	0	0	0

[1] National and regional totals exclude American Samoa, Guam, Puerto Rico, and the Virgin Islands.

Table 10
GRADUATIONS OF NURSES FROM MASTER'S PROGRAMS, BY FUNCTIONAL AREA OF STUDY: 1993-1995[1]

YEAR	TOTAL		NURSE PRACTITIONERS		ADVANCED CLINICAL PRACTICE		TEACHING		ADMINISTRATION/ MANAGEMENT		OTHER	
	Number	Percent	Number	Percent	Number	Percent	Number	Percent	Number	Percent	Number	Percent
1993	7,926	100.0	1,993	25.1	3,429	43.3	755	9.5	1,444	18.2	305	3.8
1994	8,634	100.0	2,831	32.8	3,503	40.6	854	9.9	1,446	16.7	0	0.0
1995	9,261	100.0	4,003	43.2	3,222	34.8	765	8.3	1,271	13.7	0	0.0

[1] Excludes American Samoa, Guam, Puerto Rico, and the Virgin Islands.

Table 10A
GRADUATIONS OF NURSES FROM NURSE PRACTITIONER PROGRAMS, BY NURSING CONTENT AREA: 1993-1995[1]

	1993		1994		1995	
	Number	Percent	Number	Percent	Number	Percent
Total	**1,993**	**100.0**	**2,831**	**100.0**	**4,003**	**100.0**
Adult	316	15.9	534	18.9	682	17.0
Family	705	35.4	1,073	37.9	1,511	37.7
Gerontology	137	6.9	144	5.1	179	4.5
Midwifery	184	9.2	233	8.2	292	7.3
Pediatric	276	13.8	387	13.7	431	10.8
Psych/Mental Health	64	3.2	70	2.5	95	2.4
School	26	1.3	3	0.1	8	0.2
Women's Health	115	5.8	156	5.5	231	5.8
Other	170	8.5	231	8.1	574	14.3

[1] Excludes American Samoa, Guam, Puerto Rico, and the Virgin Islands.

Table 10B
GRADUATIONS OF NURSES FROM ADVANCED CLINICAL PRACTICE, BY NURSING CONTENT AREA: 1993-1995[1]

	1993		1994		1995	
	Number	Percent	Number	Percent	Number	Percent
Total	**3,429**	**100.0**	**3,503**	**100.0**	**3,222**	**100.0**
Adult Health/Med-Surg	918	26.8	972	27.7	971	30.1
Anesthesia	187	5.5	226	6.5	273	8.5
Community Health/ Public Health	445	13.0	414	11.8	369	11.5
Critical Care	361	10.5	415	11.8	242	7.5
Gerontology/Geriatrics	168	4.9	134	3.8	181	5.6
Maternal-Child/ Parent-Child	353	10.3	319	9.1	226	7.0
Oncology	100	2.9	92	2.6	93	2.9
Pediatric	181	5.3	135	4.0	88	2.7
Psych-Mental Health	404	11.8	469	13.4	418	13.0
Other	312	9.1	327	9.3	361	11.2

[1] Excludes American Samoa, Guam, Puerto Rico, and the Virgin Islands.

Table 10C
GRADUATIONS OF NURSES FROM TEACHING, BY NURSING CONTENT AREA: 1993-1995[1]

	1993		1994		1995	
	Number	Percent	Number	Percent	Number	Percent
Total	**755**	**100.0**	**854**	**100.0**	**765**	**100.0**
Adult Health/Med-Surg	286	37.9	258	30.2	266	34.8
Anesthesia	1	0.1	16	1.9	4	0.5
Community Health/ Public Health	41	5.4	66	7.7	48	6.3
Critical Care	40	5.3	14	1.6	10	1.3
Gerontology/Geriatrics	38	5.0	18	2.1	47	6.1
Maternal-Child/ Parent-Child	57	7.5	57	6.7	12	1.6
Oncology	13	1.7	2	0.2	9	1.2
Pediatric	15	2.0	15	1.8	30	3.9
Psych-Mental Health	54	7.2	29	3.4	2	0.3
Other	210	27.8	379	44.4	337	44.0

[1] Excludes American Samoa, Guam, Puerto Rico, and the Virgin Islands.

Table 11

DOCTORAL PROGRAMS IN NURSING LOCATED IN NURSING EDUCATION DEPARTMENTS: 1986 TO 1995[1]

NLN REGION AND STATE	NUMBER OF PROGRAMS									
	1986	1987	1988	1989	1990	1991	1992	1993	1994	1995
United States	**38**	**45**	**46**	**47**	**50**	**54**	**54**	**54**	**60**	**64**
North Atlantic	10	12	12	11	11	12	12	13	16	17
Midwest	11	11	11	12	14	16	16	15	17	19
South	10	14	15	16	17	18	18	18	19	20
West	7	8	8	8	8	8	8	8	8	8
Alabama	1	1	1	1	1	1	1	1	1	1
Alaska	0	0	0	0	0	0	0	0	0	0
Arizona	1	1	1	1	1	1	1	1	1	1
Arkansas	0	0	0	0	0	0	0	0	0	0
California	2	3	3	3	3	3	3	3	3	3
Colorado	1	1	1	1	1	1	1	1	1	1
Connecticut	0	0	0	0	0	0	0	0	2	2
Delaware	0	0	0	0	0	0	0	0	0	0
District of Columbia	1	1	1	1	1	1	1	1	1	1
Florida	2	2	2	2	2	2	2	3	2	2
Georgia	1	2	2	2	2	2	2	2	2	2
Hawaii	0	0	0	0	0	0	0	0	0	0
Idaho	0	0	0	0	0	0	0	0	0	0
Illinois	2	2	2	2	3	3	3	3	3	3
Indiana	1	1	1	1	1	1	1	1	1	1
Iowa	0	0	0	1	1	1	1	1	1	1
Kansas	1	1	1	1	1	1	1	1	1	1
Kentucky	0	1	1	1	1	1	1	0	1	1
Louisiana	1	1	1	1	1	1	1	1	1	1
Maine	0	0	0	0	0	0	0	0	0	0
Maryland	1	1	1	1	1	1	1	2	2	2
Massachusetts	1	2	2	1	1	1	1	1	1	2
Michigan	2	2	2	2	2	2	2	2	2	2
Minnesota	1	1	1	1	1	1	1	1	1	1
Mississippi	0	0	0	0	0	0	0	0	0	0
Missouri	0	0	0	0	0	1	1	1	2	4
Montana	0	0	0	0	0	0	0	0	0	0
Nebraska	0	0	0	0	1	1	1	1	1	1
Nevada	0	0	0	0	0	0	0	0	0	0
New Hampshire	0	0	0	0	0	0	0	0	0	0
New Jersey	0	0	0	0	0	1	1	1	1	1
New Mexico	0	0	0	0	0	0	0	0	0	0
New York	4	5	5	5	5	5	5	6	6	6
North Carolina	0	0	1	1	1	1	1	1	1	1
North Dakota	0	0	0	0	0	0	0	0	0	0
Ohio	2	2	2	2	2	3	3	2	3	3
Oklahoma	0	0	0	0	0	0	0	0	0	0
Oregon	1	1	1	1	1	1	1	1	1	1
Pennsylvania	3	3	3	3	3	3	3	3	4	4
Rhode Island	1	1	1	1	1	1	1	1	1	1
South Carolina	0	1	1	1	1	1	1	0	1	1
South Dakota	0	0	0	0	0	0	0	0	0	0
Tennessee	0	0	0	1	2	2	2	2	2	3
Texas	2	2	2	2	2	3	3	3	3	3
Utah	1	1	1	1	1	1	1	1	1	1
Vermont	0	0	0	0	0	0	0	0	0	0
Virginia	2	3	3	3	3	3	3	3	3	3
Washington	1	1	1	1	1	1	1	1	1	1
West Virginia	0	0	0	0	0	0	0	0	0	0
Wisconsin	2	2	2	2	2	2	2	2	2	2
Wyoming	0	0	0	0	0	0	0	0	0	0
American Samoa	0	0	0	0	0	0	0	0	0	0
Guam	0	0	0	0	0	0	0	0	0	0
Puerto Rico	0	0	0	0	0	0	0	0	0	0
Virgin Islands	0	0	0	0	0	0	0	0	0	0

[1] National and regional totals exclude American Samoa, Guam, Puerto Rico, and the Virgin Islands.

[2] Due to a reanalysis, figures have been adjusted for 1991 in New York, Tennessee, the North Atlantic, the South, and the total.

Table 12
ENROLLMENTS AND PERCENTAGE CHANGE FROM PREVIOUS YEAR
OF NURSES IN DOCTORAL PROGRAMS LOCATED IN NURSING EDUCATION DEPARTMENTS:
1975 TO 1995[1]

ACADEMIC YEAR	NUMBER OF PROGRAMS	ENROLLMENTS					
		Total		Full-Time		Part-Time	
		Number	Percent Change	Number	Percent	Number	Percent
1975	12	506	+5.0	199	39.3	307	60.7
1976	14	632	+24.9	278	44.0	354	56.0
1977	16	790	+25.0	294	37.2	496	62.8
1978	21	789	-0.1	358	45.4	431	54.6
1979	22	980	+24.2	504	51.4	476	48.6
1980	22	1,019	+4.0	603	59.2	416	40.8
1981	23	1,163	+14.1	625	53.7	538	46.3
1982	25	1,342	+15.4	655	48.8	687	51.2
1983	27	1,495	+11.4	685	45.8	810	54.2
1984	31	1,696	+13.4	758	44.7	938	55.3
1985	33	1,788	+5.4	685	38.3	1,103	61.7
1986	38	1,949	+9.0	782	40.0	1,167	60.0
1987	45	2,133	+9.4	1,018	47.7	1,115	52.3
1988	46	2,309	+8.3	955	41.4	1,354	58.6
1989	47	2,417	+4.7	987	40.8	1,430	59.2
1990	50	2,504	+3.6	981	39.2	1,523	60.8
1991[2]	54	2,734	+9.2	1,157	42.3	1,577	57.7
1992	54	2,727	-0.3	1,106	40.6	1,621	59.4
1993	54	2,751	+0.9	1,092	39.7	1,662	60.4
1994	60	3,026	+10.0	1,211	40.0	1,815	60.0
1995	64	3,230	+6.7	1,357	42.0	1,873	58.0

[1] Excludes American Samoa, Guam, Puerto Rico, and the Virgin Islands.
[2] Due to a reanalysis, figures have been adjusted for 1991 for New York, Tennessee, the North Atlantic, the South, and the total.

Table 13
ENROLLMENTS OF REGISTERED NURSES IN DOCTORAL PROGRAMS LOCATED IN NURSING EDUCATION DEPARTMENTS: 1986 TO 1995[1]

NLN REGION AND STATE	NUMBER OF ENROLLMENTS									
	1986	1987	1988	1989	1990	1991	1992	1993	1994	1995
United States	**1,949**	**2,133**	**2,309**	**2,417**	**2,504**	**2,734**	**2,727**	**2,754**	**3,026**	**3,230**
North Atlantic	603	606	624	591	621	680	658	650	728	726
Midwest	426	454	530	568	645	711	774	776	795	972
South	607	716	809	836	908	915	849	866	990	1,105
West	313	357	346	422	330	428	446	462	513	427
Alabama	83	118	108	105	128	116	104	104	95	100
Alaska	0	0	0	0	0	0	0	0	0	0
Arizona	41	45	42	45	46	49	45	46	43	46
Arkansas	0	0	0	0	0	0	0	0	0	0
California	133	162	180	197	101	191	191	213	202	189
Colorado	32	37	0	39	48	57	62	59	129	45
Connecticut	0	0	0	0	0	0	0	0	14	25
Delaware	0	0	0	C	0	0	0	0	0	0
District of Columbia	71	57	62	51	47	45	48	46	42	57
Florida	44	59	67	71	81	84	86	119	94	87
Georgia	9	31	46	60	69	80	84	64	73	67
Hawaii	0	0	0	0	0	0	0	0	0	0
Idaho	0	0	0	0	0	0	0	0	0	0
Illinois	152	137	182	198	242	262	268	292	237	357
Indiana	58	56	44	50	73	57	77	69	65	68
Iowa	0	0	0	13	12	17	22	28	32	38
Kansas	23	28	29	29	23	25	26	30	31	35
Kentucky	0	10	11	15	22	24	25	0	32	31
Louisiana	17	20	32	30	45	50	72	82	88	73
Maine	0	0	0	0	0	0	0	0	0	0
Maryland	59	60	62	59	67	79	15	102	118	107
Massachusetts	44	43	38	21	31	36	38	39	46	60
Michigan	79	96	117	115	117	135	164	157	143	133
Minnesota	16	20	23	25	27	32	28	29	19	32
Mississippi	0	0	0	0	0	0	0	0	0	0
Missouri	0	0	0	0	0	17	24	30	50	79
Montana	0	0	0	0	0	0	0	0	0	0
Nebraska	0	0	0	0	8	10	14	17	17	17
Nevada	0	0	0	0	0	0	0	0	0	0
New Hampshire	0	0	0	0	0	0	0	0	0	0
New Jersey	0	0	0	0	0	15	15	19	26	31
New Mexico	0	0	0	0	0	0	0	0	0	0
New York	329	328	326	319	321	295	316	317	360	304
North Carolina	0	0	0	8	16	21	26	29	32	31
North Dakota	0	0	0	0	0	0	0	0	0	0
Ohio	76	85	94	93	93	106	103	58	131	147
Oklahoma	0	0	0	0	0	0	0	0	0	0
Oregon	18	26	36	46	40	35	47	36	30	33
Pennsylvania	148	164	178	170	188	247	204	185	191	204
Rhode Island	11	14	20	30	34	42	37	44	49	45
South Carolina	0	10	20	30	37	33	36	0	40	38
South Dakota	0	0	0	0	0	0	0	0	0	0
Tennessee	0	0	0	16	9	26	27	38	36	42
Texas	345	350	371	343	323	286	270	236	250	417
Utah	51	46	44	47	43	42	41	44	47	45
Vermont	0	0	0	0	0	0	0	0	0	0
Virginia	50	58	92	99	111	116	104	92	132	112
Washington	38	41	44	48	52	54	60	64	62	69
West Virginia	0	0	0	0	0	0	0	0	0	0
Wisconsin	22	32	41	45	50	50	48	66	70	66
Wyoming	0	0	0	0	0	0	0	0	0	0
American Samoa	0	0	0	0	0	0	0	0	0	0
Guam	0	0	0	0	0	0	0	0	0	0
Puerto Rico	0	0	0	0	0	0	0	0	0	0
Virgin Islands	0	0	0	0	0	0	0	0	0	0

[1] National and regional totals exclude American Samoa, Guam, Puerto Rico, and the Virgin Islands.

[2] Due to a reanalysis, figures have been adjusted for 1991 in New York, Tennessee, the North Atlantic, the South, and the total.

Table 14
GRADUATIONS OF REGISTERED NURSES FROM DOCTORAL PROGRAMS LOCATED IN
NURSING EDUCATION DEPARTMENTS: 1985-86 TO 1994-95[1]

NLN REGION AND STATE	NUMBER OF GRADUATIONS									
	1985-86	1986-87	1987-88	1988-89	1989-90	1990-91	1991-92	1992-93	1993-94	1994-95
United States	**249**	**257**	**284**	**324**	**295**	**355**	**391**	**381**	**373**	**425**
North Atlantic	75	80	86	88	59	71	90	99	86	92
Midwest	52	51	62	64	78	93	113	67	76	121
South	78	88	102	116	111	128	121	135	125	144
West	44	38	34	56	47	63	67	80	86	68
Alabama	11	14	18	24	16	31	19	19	28	20
Alaska	0	0	0	0	0	0	0	0	0	0
Arizona	7	7	5	7	5	4	6	10	9	6
Arkansas	0	0	0	0	0	0	0	0	0	0
California	16	10	14	23	23	37	30	33	28	33
Colorado	4	1	7	5	4	6	11	13	27	8
Connecticut	0	0	0	0	0	0	0	0	0	0
Delaware	0	0	0	0	0	0	0	0	0	0
District of Columbia	13	9	10	15	10	6	6	9	8	6
Florida	0	2	2	6	8	8	12	14	8	7
Georgia	0	0	0	0	6	3	11	10	10	7
Hawaii	0	0	0	0	0	0	0	0	0	0
Idaho	0	0	0	0	0	0	0	0	0	0
Illinois	18	16	21	21	23	33	52	24	18	40
Indiana	10	14	12	6	8	9	12	13	10	15
Iowa	0	0	0	0	0	0	4	1	2	3
Kansas	1	1	2	7	2	6	5	1	3	3
Kentucky	0	0	0	0	0	0	5	0	3	3
Louisiana	0	0	0	1	2	5	2	3	7	14
Maine	0	0	0	0	0	0	0	0	0	0
Maryland	5	5	8	8	13	7	9	6	6	11
Massachusetts	7	5	9	0	0	5	6	8	5	9
Michigan	13	8	17	10	22	18	11	8	20	23
Minnesota	0	0	1	1	2	2	6	5	4	6
Mississippi	0	0	0	0	0	0	0	0	0	0
Missouri	0	0	0	0	0	0	0	0	0	0
Montana	0	0	0	0	0	0	0	0	0	0
Nebraska	0	0	0	0	0	0	1	2	0	1
Nevada	0	0	0	0	0	0	0	0	0	0
New Hampshire	0	0	0	0	0	0	0	0	0	0
New Jersey	0	0	0	0	0	0	0	0	0	2
New Mexico	0	0	0	0	0	0	0	0	0	0
New York	46	56	51	62	30	41	46	51	41	40
North Carolina	0	0	0	0	0	0	0	0	2	3
North Dakota	0	0	0	0	0	0	0	0	0	0
Ohio	10	11	8	13	9	17	14	8	15	18
Oklahoma	0	0	0	0	0	0	0	0	0	0
Oregon	0	0	0	0	5	5	5	10	5	5
Pennsylvania	9	10	16	11	18	19	29	26	29	27
Rhode Island	0	0	0	0	1	0	3	5	3	8
South Carolina	0	0	0	0	1	7	2	0	0	6
South Dakota	0	0	0	0	0	0	0	0	0	0
Tennessee	0	0	0	0	0	0	1	4	6	4
Texas	61	65	72	71	54	56	46	57	39	45
Utah	8	12	6	10	4	3	10	5	6	5
Vermont	0	0	0	0	0	0	0	0	0	0
Virginia	1	2	2	6	11	11	14	22	16	24
Washington	9	8	2	11	6	8	5	9	11	11
West Virginia	0	0	0	0	0	0	0	0	0	0
Wisconsin	0	1	1	6	12	8	8	5	4	12
Wyoming	0	0	0	0	0	0	0	0	0	0
American Samoa	0	0	0	0	0	0	0	0	0	0
Guam	0	0	0	0	0	0	0	0	0	0
Puerto Rico	0	0	0	0	0	0	0	0	0	0
Virgin Islands	0	0	0	0	0	0	0	0	0	0

[1] National and regional totals exclude American Samoa, Guam, Puerto Rico, and the Virgin Islands.

**Section 2-4
Numeric Tables
on Male and Minority Students**

Table 1
ESTIMATED NUMBER OF ENROLLMENTS
IN MASTER'S PROGRAMS, BY RACE/ETHNICITY, NLN REGION, AND STATE: 1995[1,2]

NLN REGION AND STATE	NUMBER OF PROGRAMS	TOTAL MASTER'S ENROLLMENTS	NUMBER OF ENROLLMENTS				
			White	Black	Hispanic	Asian	American Indian
United States	**306**	**35,707**	**31,003**	**2,258**	**966**	**1,303**	**177**
North Atlantic	90	10,654	9,254	720	195	462	23
Midwest	75	9,155	8,532	361	78	144	40
South	94	10,386	8,673	975	415	262	61
West	47	5,512	4,544	202	278	435	53
Alabama	6	805	662	131	2	7	3
Alaska	1	40	40	0	0	0	0
Arizona	4	773	717	7	24	20	5
Arkansas	3	325	254	64	1	3	3
California	19	2,554	1,858	167	189	325	15
Colorado	4	480	454	7	11	6	2
Connecticut	8	712	657	29	15	11	0
Delaware	2	185	172	9	1	2	1
District of Columbia	3	291	213	55	7	16	0
Florida	9	1,397	1,084	141	102	68	2
Georgia	10	862	673	153	17	16	3
Hawaii	1	117	67	4	4	40	2
Idaho	1	22	22	0	0	0	0
Illinois	13	1,476	1,312	99	24	39	2
Indiana	9	994	928	40	9	12	5
Iowa	2	288	283	2	0	2	1
Kansas	4	531	506	11	4	7	3
Kentucky	8	448	428	7	10	1	2
Louisiana	5	321	260	50	7	3	1
Maine	3	131	130	0	0	0	1
Maryland	4	792	644	94	18	34	2
Massachusetts	11	1,530	1,442	37	20	29	2
Michigan	10	1,396	1,285	59	16	28	8
Minnesota	6	476	459	7	3	3	4
Mississippi	5	245	212	31	0	2	0
Missouri	7	873	815	44	6	7	1
Montana	1	41	38	0	0	1	2
Nebraska	3	336	333	1	1	1	0
Nevada	2	83	77	1	3	2	0
New Hampshire	2	187	185	1	0	1	0
New Jersey	8	748	663	45	15	23	2
New Mexico	2	158	132	1	21	2	2
New York	26	4,450	3,515	451	122	350	12
North Carolina	6	932	825	68	15	12	12
North Dakota	2	175	166	1	2	2	4
Ohio	10	1,672	1,551	83	5	28	5
Oklahoma	2	268	237	7	3	3	18
Oregon	2	232	213	0	6	8	5
Pennsylvania	25	2,264	2,128	89	13	29	5
Rhode Island	1	112	105	4	2	1	0
South Carolina	3	388	353	27	4	4	0
South Dakota	2	180	174	0	0	1	5
Tennessee	7	634	580	40	1	13	0
Texas	15	1,952	1,559	91	223	67	12
Utah	3	293	271	3	5	13	1
Vermont	1	44	44	0	0	0	0
Virginia	8	807	695	71	10	28	3
Washington	6	656	594	12	15	18	17
West Virginia	3	210	207	0	2	1	0
Wisconsin	7	758	720	14	8	14	2
Wyoming	1	63	61	0	0	0	2

[1] Excludes American Samoa, Guam, Puerto Rico, and the Virgin Islands.
[2] Due to rounding, the racial/ethnic estimations sometimes add up to slightly less than the true total.

113

Table 2
TRENDS IN THE ESTIMATED NUMBER OF ENROLLMENTS
OF MINORITY STUDENTS IN MASTER'S PROGRAMS, 1992-1995

YEAR	BLACKS		HISPANIC		ASIAN		AMERICAN INDIAN	
	Number	Percent	Number	Percent	Number	Percent	Number	Percent
ALL REGIONS								
1992	1,652	5.8	576	2.1	956	3.4	144	0.5
1993	1,863	6.1	758	2.5	1,056	3.5	159	0.5
1994	2,117	6.2	1,045	3.1	1,293	3.8	190	0.6
1995	2,258	6.3	966	2.7	1,303	3.7	177	0.5
NORTH ATLANTIC								
1992	467	5.6	106	1.3	411	5.0	30	0.4
1993	563	6.3	136	1.5	400	4.5	21	0.2
1994	677	6.8	238	2.4	464	4.7	26	0.3
1995	720	6.8	195	1.8	462	4.3	23	0.2
MIDWEST								
1992	303	4.4	53	0.8	115	1.7	22	0.3
1993	322	4.4	134	1.8	130	1.8	29	0.4
1994	363	4.2	72	0.8	159	1.8	45	0.5
1995	361	3.9	78	0.9	144	1.6	40	0.4
SOUTH								
1992	758	8.8	263	3.0	182	2.1	47	0.5
1993	801	8.9	307	3.4	205	2.3	58	0.6
1994	898	8.6	502	4.8	245	2.3	57	0.5
1995	975	9.4	415	4.0	262	2.5	61	0.6
WEST								
1992	124	2.7	154	3.3	248	5.4	45	1.0
1993	177	3.5	181	3.6	321	6.4	51	1.0
1994	179	3.5	233	4.6	425	8.4	62	1.2
1995	202	3.7	278	5.0	435	7.9	53	1.0

Table 3
ESTIMATED NUMBER OF GRADUATIONS
IN MASTER'S PROGRAMS, BY RACE/ETHNICITY, NLN REGION, AND STATE: 1994-1995[1,2]

NLN REGION AND STATE	NUMBER OF PROGRAMS	TOTAL MASTER'S GRADUATIONS	NUMBER OF GRADUATIONS				
			White	Black	Hispanic	Asian	American Indian
United States	**306**	**9,261**	**8,128**	**517**	**223**	**338**	**55**
North Atlantic	90	2,650	2,356	145	40	101	7
Midwest	75	2,030	1,875	73	19	46	18
South	94	2,946	2,497	245	110	79	15
West	47	1,635	1,400	54	54	112	15
Alabama	6	224	191	25	3	3	2
Alaska	1	10	9	0	1	0	0
Arizona	4	230	217	4	2	4	3
Arkansas	3	65	56	7	0	2	0
California	19	755	599	43	34	74	5
Colorado	4	139	130	3	6	0	0
Connecticut	8	151	142	3	1	5	0
Delaware	2	53	49	2	2	0	0
District of Columbia	3	109	78	19	6	6	0
Florida	9	321	242	34	28	16	1
Georgia	10	232	190	34	3	5	0
Hawaii	1	36	23	0	0	13	0
Idaho	1	27	20	0	3	2	2
Illinois	13	375	333	21	5	9	7
Indiana	9	182	159	11	4	8	0
Iowa	2	50	48	0	0	1	1
Kansas	4	127	118	2	3	4	0
Kentucky	8	71	69	0	1	1	0
Louisiana	5	113	90	21	1	1	0
Maine	3	19	18	0	0	0	1
Maryland	4	205	171	13	5	16	0
Massachusetts	11	433	412	9	3	8	0
Michigan	10	234	217	12	2	4	0
Minnesota	6	133	130	0	1	1	1
Mississippi	5	112	95	9	6	2	0
Missouri	7	177	168	5	0	2	2
Montana	1	5	5	0	0	0	0
Nebraska	3	50	48	1	1	0	0
Nevada	2	10	9	0	0	0	1
New Hampshire	2	27	27	0	0	0	0
New Jersey	8	110	95	4	2	9	0
New Mexico	2	37	33	1	2	0	1
New York	26	1,113	928	90	26	63	6
North Carolina	6	235	215	16	0	3	1
North Dakota	2	49	44	0	0	0	5
Ohio	10	459	428	19	1	10	1
Oklahoma	2	49	44	2	1	0	2
Oregon	2	121	113	0	1	6	1
Pennsylvania	25	607	579	18	0	10	0
Rhode Island	1	26	26	0	0	0	0
South Carolina	3	116	99	11	2	4	0
South Dakota	2	24	23	0	0	0	1
Tennessee	7	330	293	22	11	2	2
Texas	15	564	463	29	43	22	7
Utah	3	82	77	0	1	4	0
Vermont	1	2	2	0	0	0	0
Virginia	8	269	241	22	5	1	0
Washington	6	171	154	3	3	9	2
West Virginia	3	40	38	0	1	1	0
Wisconsin	7	170	159	2	2	7	0
Wyoming	1	12	11	0	1	0	0

[1] Excludes American Samoa, Guam, Puerto Rico, and the Virgin Islands.
[2] Due to rounding, the racial/ethnic estimations sometimes add up to slightly less than the true total.

Table 4
TRENDS IN THE ESTIMATED NUMBER OF GRADUATIONS
OF MINORITY STUDENTS FROM MASTER'S PROGRAMS, 1991-92 TO 1994-95

YEAR	BLACKS Number	BLACKS Percent	HISPANIC Number	HISPANIC Percent	ASIAN Number	ASIAN Percent	AMERICAN INDIAN Number	AMERICAN INDIAN Percent
ALL REGIONS								
1991-92	400	5.4	115	1.6	250	3.4	29	0.4
1992-93	440	5.6	158	2.0	262	3.3	40	0.5
1993-94	517	6.0	282	3.3	274	3.2	44	0.5
1994-95	517	5.6	223	2.4	338	3.6	55	0.6
NORTH ATLANTIC								
1991-92	138	6.1	30	1.3	88	3.9	8	0.4
1992-93	118	5.1	25	1.1	63	2.7	11	0.5
1993-94	144	6.0	43	1.8	98	4.1	6	0.2
1994-95	145	5.5	40	1.5	101	3.8	7	0.3
MIDWEST								
1991-92	66	4.0	13	0.8	40	2.4	4	0.2
1992-93	72	4.0	27	1.5	41	2.3	4	0.2
1993-94	85	4.5	18	1.0	37	2.0	8	0.4
1994-95	73	3.6	19	0.9	46	2.3	18	0.9
SOUTH								
1991-92	165	7.6	42	1.9	54	2.5	8	0.4
1992-93	204	8.6	59	2.5	73	3.1	9	0.4
1993-94	228	8.2	165	6.0	50	1.8	17	0.6
1994-95	245	8.3	110	3.7	79	2.7	15	0.5
WEST								
1991-92	31	2.4	30	2.4	68	5.4	9	0.7
1992-93	46	3.3	47	3.4	85	6.2	16	1.2
1993-94	60	3.8	56	3.6	89	5.7	13	0.8
1994-95	54	3.3	54	3.3	112	6.9	15	0.9

Table 5
NUMBER OF ENROLLMENTS OF MALE STUDENTS
IN MASTER'S PROGRAMS, BY NLN REGION: 1995[1]

	NUMBER OF REPORTING PROGRAMS	TOTAL ENROLLMENTS	MALES	
			Number	Percent
All Regions	**250**	**32,969**	**1,954**	**5.9**
North Atlantic	73	9,782	469	4.8
Midwest	57	7,940	368	4.6
South	76	9,782	710	7.3
West	44	5,465	407	7.4

[1] Excludes American Samoa, Guam, Puerto Rico, and the Virgin Islands.

Table 6
NUMBER OF GRADUATIONS OF MALE STUDENTS
FROM MASTER'S PROGRAMS, BY NLN REGION: 1994-95[1]

	NUMBER OF REPORTING PROGRAMS	TOTAL GRADUATIONS	MALES	
			Number	Percent
All Regions	**140**	**6,964**	**435**	**6.2**
North Atlantic	38	1,948	97	5.0
Midwest	35	1,572	77	4.9
South	40	2,130	163	7.7
West	27	1,314	98	7.5

[1] Excludes American Samoa, Guam, Puerto Rico, and the Virgin Islands.

PART THREE
FOCUS ON PRACTICAL/
VOCATIONAL NURSING

Section 3-1
Executive Summary

EXECUTIVE SUMMARY

According to the results from the 1995 NLN Annual Survey of PN/VN programs, the number of programs remained unchanged at 1,107 (Figure 1). The number of adult programs (1,107) increased by 23, while the number of high school extended programs (68) increased by 3 percent and high school programs remained at 35 (Figure 2).

The Southern region continued to record the highest number of programs (505) followed by the Midwest (25). The North Atlantic had 176 programs while the West had the least (168). By state, Texas had the highest number of programs (104) and Rhode Island had the lowest (1). Alaska continued to report no LPN/LVN programs.

Publicly funded programs decreased in number but still accounted for more than 90 percent of the total programs (Figure 3). Privately run programs continued to increase and reached a record number of programs (95). Most programs, both public and private, were located in the South. The decrease in public programs was evident across all regions except the Midwest which showed a slight increase reaching 246 (Figure 4).

ADMISSIONS, ENROLLMENTS AND GRADUATIONS

Annual admissions of new students to LPN/LVN programs declined in 1995; total admissions were 57,906, a change of 4.5 percent (Figure 5). This decline occurred in all regions of the country. There was an overall increase in the number of annual admissions within private institutions but a decrease within public institutions. This decline was also evident in diploma and associate degree programs; however, baccalaureate degree programs showed a small increase in annual admissions (Figure 6).

Fall admissions (34,733) continued on a two year decline (Figure 7). The number of fall admissions declined in all regions, but most significantly in the West. The decline in fall admissions was evident across all RN program types and represented a 7.5 percent change from 1994 (Figure 8).

Enrollments in LPN/LVN programs (56,028) continued on a downward trend for the second consecutive year, a percentage change of 5.7 from 1994 (Figure 9). All regions of the country experienced such a decline; the South had the highest enrollment (25, 503) and the West the lowest (6,343). Texas has become the state with the highest enrollments at 4,902, and some states reported no enrollments.

Privately supported institutions showed an increase in enrollment across all regions but there was a 7 percent decline in enrollment in the publicly supported programs. All types of administratively controlled programs except senior colleges or universities and independent agencies showed a decline in their enrollment of LPN/LVN students.

A downward trend in enrollments for the 1995 year was also evident across all RN program types. The overall number of students enrolled in RN programs dropped by 2.7 percent for diploma, associate, and baccalaureate degree programs combined (Figure 10). This was the first recorded decline in enrollments for baccalaureate degree programs since 1988.

The number of students graduating from LPN/LVN programs in 1995 (44,234) decreased by 1.9 percent (Figure 11). There was a decline in all regions except the South which reported a small increase. By state, programs in Texas had the highest number of LPN/LVN graduates (4,503). Privately controlled schools had an increase in the number of graduates and public schools had a decrease. By administrative control, technical or vocational schools had the highest number of graduates but still experienced a decrease in the number of graduates overall.

The trend of declining graduations in LPN/LVN programs was also evident in associate degree and diploma programs by less than 1 percent. There was, however, an increase of 8.1 percent in the number of graduates from basic baccalaureate programs, resulting in an overall increase in graduations from RN programs by 2.3 percent (Figure 12).

Tuition for LPN/LVN programs overall continues to be lower than tuition rates for RN programs. Mean annual tuition for LPN/LVN programs increased in private institutions to $5,834, a 26.6 percent increase. Public institutions also increased tuition for residents but decreased tuition by a small margin for non-residents. Among RN programs the average annual tuition at public institutions was $1,984 for state resident and $4,973 for non-residents, a 13 percent increase from 1994-95. At private institutions the average annual tuition was $7,970 among all RN programs.

DEMAND FOR ENTRY TO LPN/LVN PROGRAMS

The number of applications to LPN/LVN programs dropped significantly in 1995 to 70,085, an 18 percent decrease. The number of applications per fall admissions were 2.58, a decrease from the 1994 figure of 3.02. Of those applying for admission, 41.1 percent were accepted and 17 percent were placed on a waiting list.

MEN AND MINORITIES

Fewer men were admitted to LPN/LVN programs in 1995, a 1.1 percent difference from the previous year (Figure 13). Simultaneously, the number of men enrolled in these programs also decreased from 12.6 percent in 1994 to 11.6 percent in 1995. The same trend continued for graduations where there was a nominal decline of 0.2 percent. Almost 51 percent of all men enrolled in LPN/LVN programs were from programs located in the South. Graduation of men from LPN/LVN programs also showed a slight decline of 0.2 percent, representing 12.6 percent of all graduates.

About 32 percent of all LPN/LVNs admitted were minority students, an increase of 7.2 percent from 1994. The largest minority group admitted were blacks (20.9%) followed by Hispanics (6.1%), Asians (3.5%), and American Indians (1.6%). The highest percentage of minority students admitted (47%) was in the Western region and the lowest (22.4%) was in the Midwest.

Minority enrollment increased overall in 1995, representing 29.9 percent of the enrollment pool, an increase of 2.1 percent from 1994 (Figure 14). The highest minority representation was among blacks (18.7%). Hispanic and American Indian enrollment continued to increase reaching 6.3 percent and 1.8 percent respectively. Asian enrollment remained unchanged at 3.1 percent from the previous year.

Graduates from minority groups totaled 26.2 percent of the graduating class of 1995. Most of the minority graduates were blacks (15.7%), followed by Hispanics (5.5%), Asians (3.5%) and American Indians (1.5%). The region recording the largest percentage of minority graduates was the West at 35.9 percent and the lowest was in the Midwest at 17.7 percent.

RESULTS OF SUPPLEMENTARY QUESTIONS
INCLUDED IN THE 1995 LPN/LVN SURVEY

Several new questions were included in the 1995 Annual Survey of LPN/LVN programs that reflect the current issues in nursing education. These questions addressed issues surrounding involvement in international education and interdisciplinary programs.

With respect to international education, very few LPN/LVN programs reported any faculty to faculty exchange (2.9%) and even fewer schools reported any study abroad program for students (0.8%). Only 0.9 percent of LPN/LVN programs reported that they were involved in some kind of collaborative research/teaching/training program with international agencies or universities. Another 1.7 percent indicated that they had some kind of collaborative agreement through non-governmental organizations.

Less than one-fourth of LPN/LVN programs participated in any type of interdisciplinary programs (Figure 15). Most programs surveyed reported that nursing faculty taught interdisciplinary courses (23.2%). A slightly lower number (20.5%) indicated that nursing faculty participated in the development of some kind of interdisciplinary faculty practices. Less than one-fifth (15.4%) participated in the regional accreditation of colleges and only 3.5 percent had nursing faculty serving on a dissertation committee for students from other disciplines. Of all the schools responding, 7.2 percent reported that faculty were preparing research grants with faculty from other disciplines.

When asked about the settings used by nursing students for their clinical experience, most of the experience was gained in acute care settings as reported by 34 percent of the programs. The majority of the schools indicated that students spent less than 20 percent of their time in community based care settings. Close to 35 percent of the schools indicated that less than 40 percent of the student's time was spent in long-term care settings.

The use of computers in schools was another issue addressed in this year's survey. Less than half of all schools (45.4%) said that they used MS-DOS as their application software and 46.2 percent used Windows. Only 9.2 percent reported using Macintosh hardware compared to 47.4 percent using PCs and 5.2 percent using Mainframe computers.

Less than one-third of all LPN/LVN programs reported an intention to reduce the number of students admitted to their programs (Figure 16). The most common reason cited for the reduction in admissions is lack of perceived job opportunities (19.1%). Budget reductions was the second most common reason cited for reductions in LPN/LVN programs (10.5%) followed by the lack of qualified applicants (7.1%). The estimated percentage of the reduction was less than 20 percent for most schools (14.2%), and another 11.1 percent of the programs intended to reduce enrollment by 21 to 40 percent of the current class.

SUMMARY

Several trends seem to be evident from the results of the LPN/LVN survey of 1995. There was no change in the number of programs; there was clearly a decline in annual admissions, enrollments and graduations. The number of Fall admissions, which is a predictor of future enrollment was also on the decline.

This trend has continued across RN programs where we see an overall decline in enrollment, fall admissions, and the number of applications to RN programs. This is not a complete surprise since LPN/LVNs generally continue their education in other programs, particularly diploma and associate degree programs. The decline in LPN/LVN enrollment may affect RN enrollment further, some time in the future, and may indicate a trickle down effect since LPN/LVNs make up a significant proportion of those students applying to RN programs.

The decline in the number of students enrolled may be partially due to the perception both from nursing program administrators and students of an impending shortage of job opportunities. Also, because of the lack of funds available to nursing programs, schools are reducing the number of students they admit to their programs. We must be vigilant in observing whether this trend continues or if this is a temporary trend due to the current climate in the health care industry, as these have obvious implications for recruitment, education and service delivery.

Sherlene Trotman, MS
Research Coordinator
NLN Center for Research in Nursing
 Education and Community Health

Delroy Louden, PhD
Executive Director
NLN Center for Research in Nursing
 Education and Community Health

Section 3-2
Graphs

FIGURE 1
LPN/LVN PROGRAMS REMAIN STAGNANT

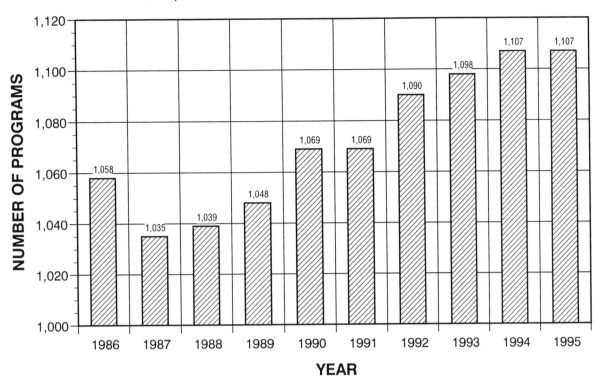

FIGURE 2
ADULT PROGRAMS INCREASED BY 23

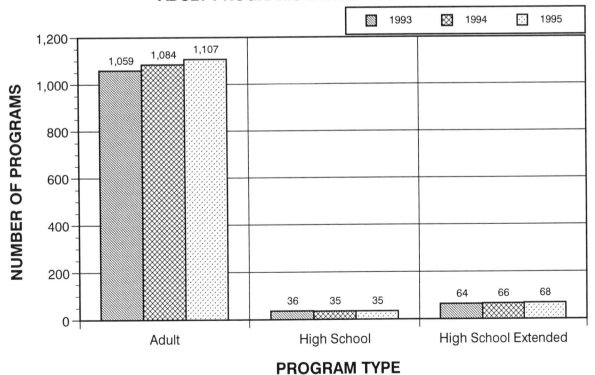

FIGURE 3
NUMBER OF PUBLIC PROGRAMS DECREASED,
WHILE PRIVATE PROGRAMS INCREASED

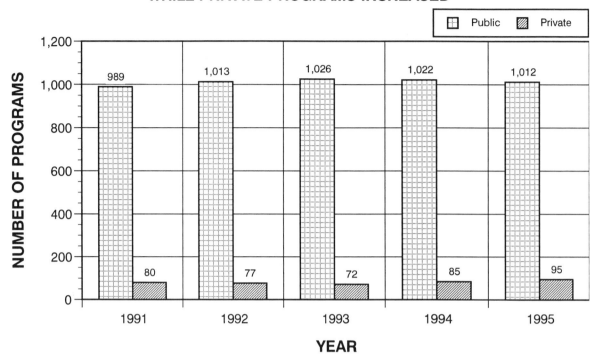

FIGURE 4
MOST PROGRAMS, BOTH PUBLIC AND PRIVATE LOCATED IN THE SOUTH

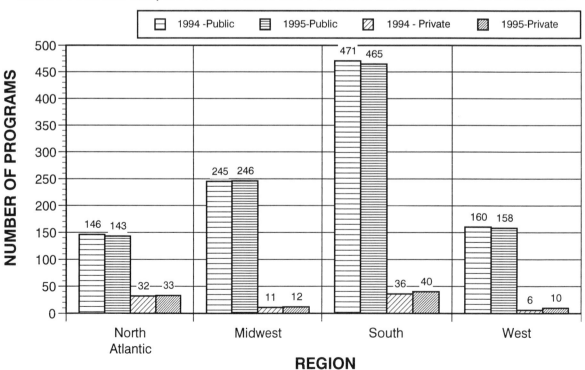

FIGURE 5
ANNUAL ADMISSIONS EXPERIENCED A MAJOR DECLINE

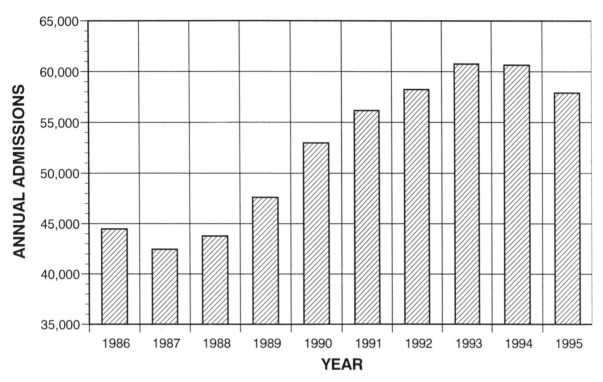

FIGURE 6
DECLINE IN LPN/LVN ANNUAL ADMISSIONS
ALSO EVIDENT IN DIPLOMA AND ASSOCIATE DEGREE PROGRAMS

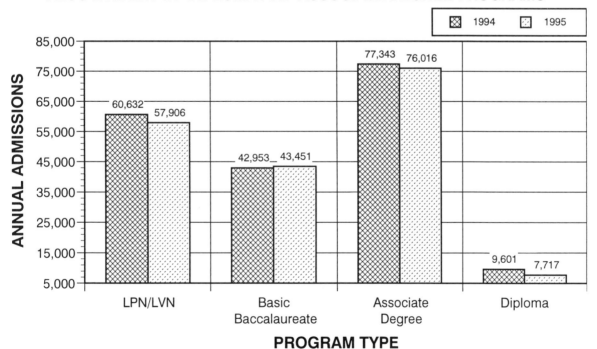

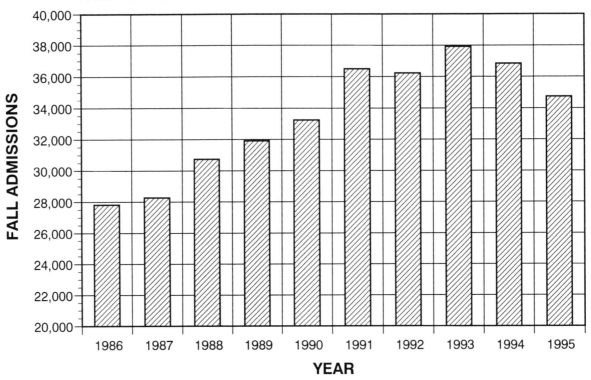

FIGURE 7
FALL ADMISSIONS DROPPED BY MORE THAN 5 PERCENT

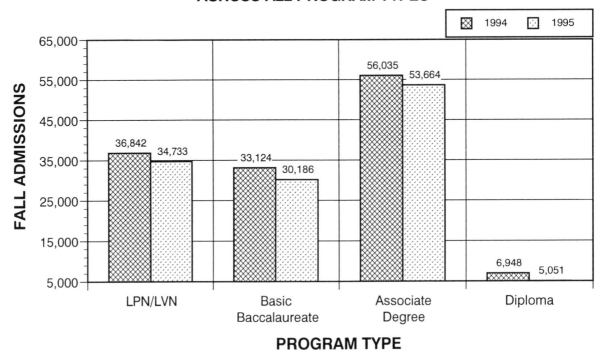

FIGURE 8
DECLINE IN FALL ADMISSIONS EVIDENT
ACROSS ALL PROGRAM TYPES

FIGURE 9
ENROLLMENTS DECLINED FOR THE SECOND CONSECUTIVE YEAR

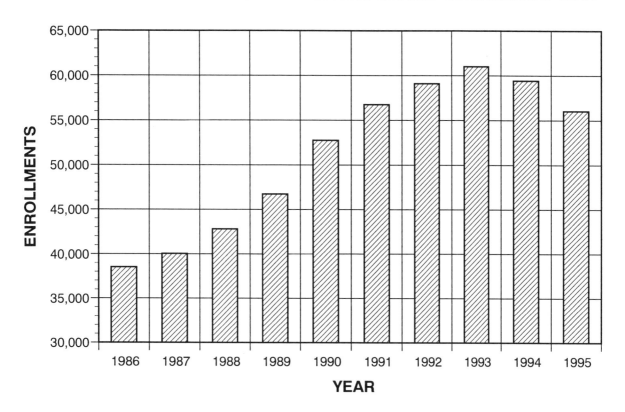

FIGURE 10
ENROLLMENTS IN NURSING PROGRAMS EXPERIENCED
DOWNWARD TREND ACROSS ALL PROGRAM TYPES

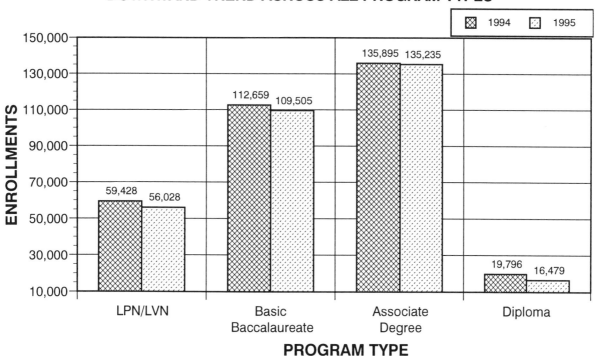

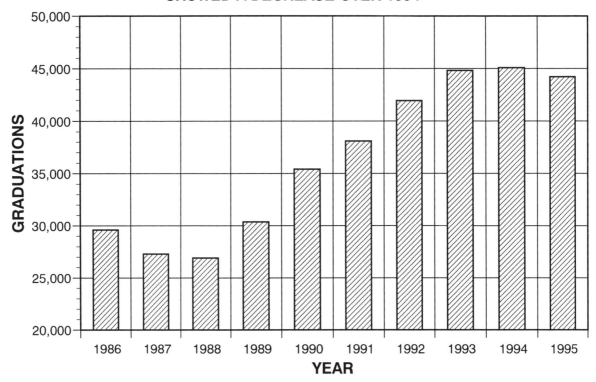

FIGURE 11
1995 LPN/LVN GRADUATIONS
SHOWED A DECREASE OVER 1994

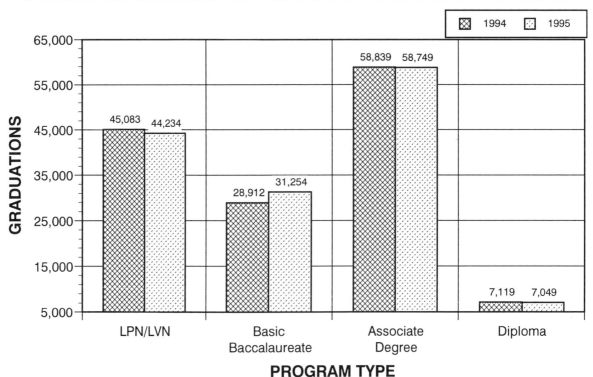

FIGURE 12
GRADUATIONS INCREASED ONLY IN BASIC BACCALAUREATE PROGRAMS

134

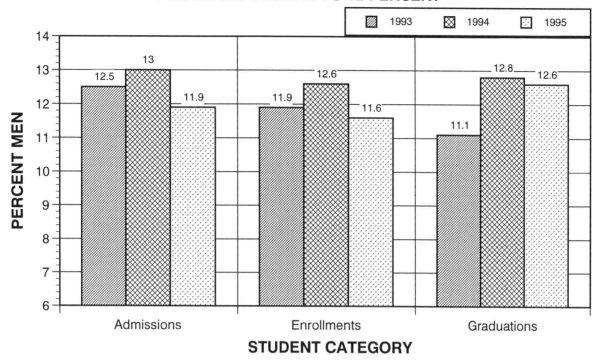

FIGURE 13
PERCENTAGE OF MEN IN LPN/LVN
PROGRAMS DECLINE TO 12 PERCENT

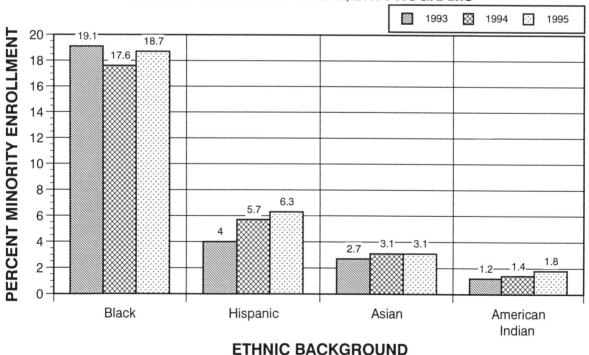

FIGURE 14
INCREASE IN PERCENTAGE OF BLACK
STUDENTS ENROLLED IN LPN/LVN PROGRAMS

FIGURE 15
LESS THAN ONE FOURTH OF LPN/LVN PROGRAMS PARTICIPATE IN INTERDISCIPLINARY PROGRAMS

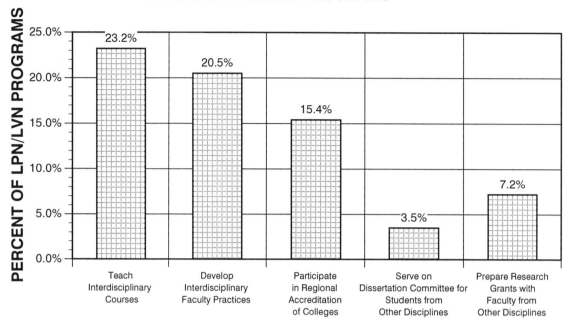

FIGURE 16
WHY LPN/LVN PROGRAMS REDUCE ADMISSIONS

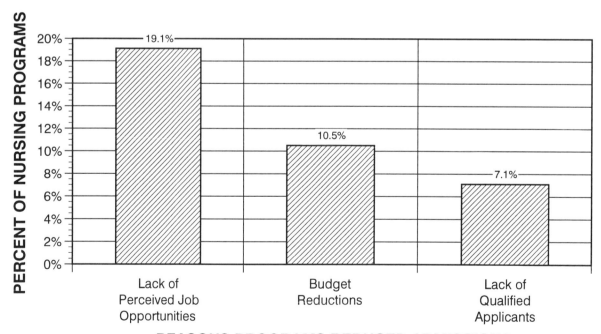

Section 3-3
Numeric Tables

Table 1
LPN/LVN SCHOOLS AND PROGRAMS
WITH PERCENTAGE CHANGE FROM PREVIOUS YEAR, BY TYPE OF PROGRAM: 1976 TO 1995

YEAR[1]	SCHOOLS[2]		All L.P.N./L.V.N. Programs		Adult Programs[3]		High School Programs[4]		High School Extended Programs[5]	
	Number	Percent Change	Number	Percent Change	Number	Percent Change	Number	Percent Change	Number	Percent Change
1976	1,236	+0.6	1,318	+0.2	1,155	-0.1	66	+4.8	97	+1.0
1977	1,234	-0.2	1,319	+0.1	1,155	+0.0	63	-4.5	101	+4.1
1978	1,232	-0.2	1,310	-0.7	1,156	+0.1	60	-4.8	94	-6.9
1979	1,222	-0.8	1,298	-0.9	1,147	-0.8	60	+0.0	91	-3.2
1980	1,221	-0.1	1,299	+0.1	1,153	+0.5	55	-8.3	91	+0.0
1981	1,231	+0.8	1,309	+0.8	1,163	+0.9	55	+0.0	91	+0.0
1982	1,221	-0.8	1,295	-1.1	1,153	-0.9	55	+0.0	91	+0.0
1983	1,218	-0.2	1,297	+0.2	1,154	+0.1	56	+0.0	87	-4.4
1984	1,162	-4.6	1,254	-3.3	1,114	-3.5	57	+1.8	83	-4.6
1985	1,128	-2.9	1,165	-7.1	1,048	-5.9	50	-12.3	67	-19.3
1986	1,058	-6.2	1,087	-6.7	947	-38.3	53	+6.0	58	-13.4
1987	1,035	-2.2	1,068	-1.7	922	-2.6	47	-17.5	66	+13.8
1988	1,039	-2.7	1,095	+0.4	989	+7.3	44	-6.4	62	-6.1
1989	1,048	+0.9	1,171	+6.9	1,050	+6.2	47	+6.8	74	+19.4
1990	1,069	+2.0	1,154[6]	-1.4	1,023	-2.6	46	-2.1	85	+14.9
1991	1,069	+0.0	1,125	-2.5	1,024	+0.1	40	-15.0	61	-28.8
1992	1,090	+2.0	1,154	+2.6	1,053	+2.8	42	+5.0	59	-3.3
1993	1,098	+0.7	1,159	+0.4	1,059	+0.6	36	-14.3	64	+8.5
1994	1,107	+0.8	1,185[1]	+2.2	1,084	+2.4	35	-2.8	66	+3.1
1995	1,107	+0.0	1,210	+2.1	1,107	+2.1	35	+0.0	68	+3.0

[1] As of October 15.

[2] Excludes American Samoa, Guam, Puerto Rico, and the Virgin Islands.

[3] Adult programs are conducted primarily for adults and out-of-school youth and have not been planned as part of a high school curriculum.

[4] High School programs are conducted primarily for high school students and lead concurrently to a high school diploma and eligibility for writing the licensure examination.

[5] High School Extended programs are conducted primarily for high school students and lead to a high school diploma, but require some additional months of preparation after high school graduation.

[6] This decline in the number of LPN/LVN programs can be partially attributed to two major trends. The consolidation of some programs and the temporary suspension of others.

Table 2
LPN/LVN PROGRAMS, BY NLN REGION AND STATE: 1986 TO 1995

NLN REGION AND STATE	NUMBER OF PROGRAMS									
	1986	1987	1988	1989	1990	1991	1992	1993	1994	1995
United States[1]	**1,058**	**1,035**	**1,039**	**1,048**	**1,069**	**1,069**	**1,090**	**1,098**	**1,107**	**1,107**
North Atlantic	192	180	179	180	183	177	179	177	178	176
Midwestern	235	233	232	236	242	245	252	254	256	258
Southern	459	451	461	468	483	485	494	501	507	505
Western	172	171	167	164	161	162	165	166	166	168
Alabama	22	22	22	22	23	23	23	22	22	22
Alaska	0	0	0	0	0	0	0	0	0	0
Arizona	10	10	9	9	10	11	13	13	13	13
Arkansas	27	28	27	27	27	27	27	27	29	28
California	76	78	75	73	68	67	68	69	67	69
Colorado	14	14	14	14	15	15	15	15	17	17
Connecticut	11	11	11	11	11	11	12	12	13	12
Delaware	3	3	3	3	3	3	3	3	3	3
District of Columbia	2	2	2	2	3	3	3	3	3	3
Florida	34	34	34	36	39	39	40	41	42	41
Georgia	41	40	40	41	39	37	37	38	38	38
Hawaii	4	4	4	4	4	4	4	4	4	4
Idaho	6	5	5	5	5	5	5	5	5	5
Illinois	32	31	30	32	32	32	35	36	36	36
Indiana	17	18	19	19	21	21	21	22	22	22
Iowa	25	25	25	25	26	26	26	26	26	26
Kansas	16	16	16	16	17	17	17	17	17	17
Kentucky	17	17	17	17	18	18	18	17	17	17
Louisiana	35	35	35	34	39	39	40	45	46	45
Maine	5	5	5	5	5	5	5	5	5	5
Maryland	14	14	14	15	15	14	14	11	13	11
Massachusetts	22	22	22	21	22	20	20	20	20	20
Michigan	27	27	26	26	28	28	27	27	27	27
Minnesota	26	26	26	26	26	27	25	25	24	24
Mississippi	12	13	13	14	14	13	14	15	15	15
Missouri	32	31	31	32	33	34	36	36	38	39
Montana	5	5	5	5	5	5	5	5	5	5
Nebraska	8	8	8	9	7	7	7	7	7	7
Nevada	4	3	3	3	2	2	2	2	2	2
New Hampshire	4	3	3	2	2	2	2	2	2	2
New Jersey	31	26	25	25	25	25	26	25	24	23
New Mexico	8	7	7	7	7	8	8	8	8	8
New York	60	57	56	57	57	53	53	53	54	54
North Carolina	24	23	23	27	28	31	32	32	32	31
North Dakota	3	3	3	3	3	4	5	5	5	6
Ohio	41	42	41	41	40	40	40	40	41	41
Oklahoma	25	25	27	27	29	29	29	30	28	30
Oregon	11	11	11	10	11	11	11	11	11	11
Pennsylvania	50	47	48	50	51	51	51	50	50	50
Rhode Island	1	1	1	1	1	1	1	1	1	1
South Carolina	20	20	21	21	21	21	21	23	23	23
South Dakota	1	1	1	2	2	2	2	2	2	2
Tennessee	20	22	23	22	22	25	28	27	28	26
Texas	100	91	98	97	100	100	102	103	103	104
Utah	6	6	6	6	6	6	6	6	6	6
Vermont	3	3	3	3	3	3	3	3	3	3
Virginia	49	48	48	49	49	49	49	49	50	53
Washington	22	22	22	22	22	22	22	22	22	22
West Virginia	19	19	19	19	20	20	20	21	21	21
Wisconsin	7	5	6	5	7	7	11	11	11	11
Wyoming	6	6	6	6	6	6	6	6	6	6
American Samoa	1	1	1	1	1	1	1	1	1	2
Guam	0	0	0	0	0	0	0	0	0	0
Puerto Rico	24	24	21	21	25	26	26	25	40	43
Virgin Islands	0	0	1	1	1	2	2	2	2	2

[1] National and regional totals exclude American Samoa, Guam, Puerto Rico, and the Virgin Islands.

Table 3
LPN/LVN PROGRAMS, BY NLN REGION AND PRIMARY SOURCE OF FINANCIAL SUPPORT: 1986 TO 1995

NLN REGION BY TYPE OF FINANCIAL SUPPORT[1]	NUMBER OF PROGRAMS									
	1986	1987	1988	1989	1990	1991	1992	1993	1994	1995
All Regions	**1,058**	**1,035**	**1,039**	**1,048**	**1,069**	**1,069**	**1,090**	**1,098**	**1,107**	**1,107**
Public	986	958	962	976	985	989	1,013	1,026	1,022	1,012
Private	72	77	77	72	84	80	77	72	85	95
North Atlantic	192	180	179	180	183	179	179	177	178	176
Public	162	152	150	154	152	146	147	149	146	143
Private	30	28	29	26	31	31	32	28	32	33
Midwest	235	233	232	236	242	245	252	254	256	258
Public	225	220	224	226	229	235	244	246	245	246
Private	10	13	8	10	13	10	8	8	11	12
South	459	451	461	468	483	485	494	501	507	505
Public	436	425	431	439	448	450	460	469	471	465
Private	23	26	30	29	35	35	34	32	36	40
West	172	171	167	164	161	162	165	166	166	168
Public	163	161	157	157	156	158	162	162	160	158
Private	9	10	10	7	5	4	3	4	6	10

[1] Excludes American Samoa, Guam, Puerto Rico, and the Virgin Islands.

Table 4A
ADMINISTRATIVE CONTROL BY REGION, 1995[1]

	NORTH ATLANTIC	MIDWEST	SOUTH	WEST	ALL REGIONS
Administrative Control					
Technical or Vocational School	69.3	46.1	52.3	22.0	49.0
Junior or Community College	11.9	45.7	34.3	67.9	38.5
Secondary School	8.5	6 .2	6.5	6.5	6.8
Hospital	7.4	0.8	5.0	0.6	3.7
Government Agency	0.6	0.0	0.2	1.2	0.4
Senior College or University	0.6	1.2	1.0	1.8	1.1
Independent Agency	1 .7	0.0	0.8	0.0	0.6

[1] Excludes American Samoa, Guam, Puerto Rico, and the Virgin Islands.

Table 4B

LPN/LVN PROGRAMS, BY NLN REGION AND TYPE OF ADMINISTRATIVE CONTROL: 1986 TO 1995

NLN REGION BY TYPE OF ADMINISTRATIVE CONTROL [1]	NUMBER OF PROGRAMS									
	1986	1987	1988	1989	1990	1991	1992	1993	1994	1995
All Regions	**1,058**	**1,035**	**1,039**	**1,048**	**1,069**	**1,069**	**1,090**	**1,098**	**1,107**	**1,107**
Technical or vocational school	554	538	526	513	532	532	546	547	550	542
Junior or community college	354	362	384	397	404	414	407	417	426	426
Secondary school	80	71	67	70	65	63	73	70	69	75
Hospital	45	40	45	47	49	39	41	39	41	41
Government agency	6	13	8	9	9	9	5	5	5	4
Senior college or university	10	5	5	7	6	8	12	13	10	12
Independent agency	9	6	4	3	4	4	6	7	6	7
North Atlantic	192	180	179	180	183	177	179	177	178	176
Technical or vocational school	126	115	118	113	121	118	119	116	121	122
Junior or community college	20	19	19	23	22	24	24	26	23	21
Secondary school	26	27	24	25	21	17	17	16	17	15
Hospital	15	13	15	15	15	13	13	12	13	13
Government agency	2	5	3	3	3	3	2	3	2	1
Senior college or university	0	0	0	1	1	2	3	3	1	1
Independent agency	3	1	0	0	0	0	1	1	1	3
Midwest	235	233	232	236	242	245	252	254	256	258
Technical or vocational school	118	118	112	110	118	126	125	125	125	119
Junior or community college	99	99	105	108	109	106	110	112	117	118
Secondary school	12	10	9	11	8	7	12	11	9	16
Hospital	3	3	3	3	3	2	2	2	1	2
Government agency	0	1	1	1	2	2	0	0	1	0
Senior college or university	2	1	1	2	1	1	2	2	2	3
Independent agency	1	1	1	1	1	1	1	2	1	0
South	459	451	461	468	483	485	494	501	507	505
Technical or vocational school	261	258	255	253	256	256	265	268	268	264
Junior or community college	128	132	149	156	164	172	162	167	172	173
Secondary school	32	26	23	23	26	26	32	32	32	33
Hospital	27	24	27	29	30	24	26	24	26	25
Government agency	4	7	3	4	3	3	2	1	1	1
Senior college or university	3	2	2	2	2	2	4	5	5	5
Independent agency	4	2	2	1	2	2	3	4	3	4
West	172	171	167	164	161	162	165	166	166	168
Technical or vocational school	49	47	41	39	37	32	37	38	36	37
Junior or community college	107	112	111	110	109	112	111	112	114	114
Secondary school	10	8	11	11	10	13	12	11	11	11
Hospital	0	0	0	0	1	0	0	1	1	1
Government agency	0	0	1	1	1	1	1	1	1	2
Senior college or university	5	2	2	2	2	3	3	3	2	3
Independent agency	1	2	1	1	1	1	1	0	1	0

[1] Excludes American Samoa, Guam, Puerto Rico, and the Virgin Islands.

Table 5
ADMISSIONS TO LPN/LVN PROGRAMS
AND PERCENTAGE CHANGE FROM PREVIOUS YEAR:
1975-76 TO 1994-95

| YEAR[1] | ADMISSIONS TO LPN/LVN PROGRAMS | |
	Number[2]	Percent Change
1975-76	61,353	+1.7
1976-77	60,166	-1.9
1977-78	60,610	+0.7
1978-79	57,081	-5.8
1979-80	56,316	-1.3
1980-81	58,479	+3.8
1981-82	60,426	+3.3
1982-83	61,453	+1.7
1983-84	57,865	-5.8
1984-85	47,034	-18.7
1985-86	44,477	-5.4
1986-87	42,452	-4.6
1987-88	43,774	+3.0
1988-89	47,602	+8.8
1989-90	52,969	+11.3
1990-91	56,176	+5.7
1991-92	58,245	+3.7
1992-93	60,749	+4.3
1993-94	60,632	-0.2
1994-95	57,906	-4.5

[1] Time period is August 1 through July 31.
[2] Excludes American Samoa, Guam, Puerto Rico, and the Virgin Islands.

Table 6
ANNUAL ADMISSIONS TO LPN/LVN PROGRAMS, BY NLN REGION AND STATE: 1985-86 TO 1994-95

NLN REGION AND STATE	NUMBER OF ADMISSIONS									
	1985-86	1986-87	1987-88	1988-89	1989-90	1990-91	1991-92	1992-93	1993-94	1994-95
United States[1]	**44,477**	**42,452**	**43,774**	**47,602**	**52,969**	**56,176**	**58,245**	**60,749**	**60,632**	**57,906**
North Atlantic	9,332	7,789	7,985	8,972	10,558	10,653	11,156	11,896	11,986	10,969
Midwest	9,556	10,145	10,256	11,332	12,802	13,857	13,534	14,115	14,580	13,145
South	18,404	17,779	19,073	21,087	22,743	25,049	26,365	27,544	27,956	27,400
West	7,185	6,739	6,460	6,211	6,866	6,617	7,190	7,194	6,110	6,392
Alabama	1,345	1,304	1,517	1,909	2,207	2,405	3,126	3,082	3,372	3,117
Alaska	0	0	0	0	0	0	0	0	0	0
Arizona	338	380	403	342	468	434	387	388	408	337
Arkansas	691	755	771	870	766	1,002	1,007	964	898	1,016
California	3,830	3,372	3,658	3,538	3,736	3,987	4,366	4,600	3,152	3,580
Colorado	302	466	333	407	424	362	547	354	481	442
Connecticut	425	335	319	428	455	410	461	476	469	442
Delaware	88	99	116	113	110	109	108	80	124	165
District of Columbia	277	159	283	107	277	212	203	160	145	256
Florida	2,218	2,212	2,343	2,710	2,968	3,353	3,478	3,300	3,560	3,555
Georgia	1,708	1,581	1,412	1,900	1,927	2,081	2,124	2,369	2,344	2,278
Hawaii	141	109	112	110	173	92	112	58	128	178
Idaho	137	107	119	139	141	160	152	158	160	160
Illinois	1,585	1,728	1,540	1,662	1,960	1,948	1,936	1,967	2,151	2,053
Indiana	862	932	1,078	1,170	1,407	1,493	1,665	1,769	1,859	1,726
Iowa	607	1,007	771	930	1,243	1,008	1,067	970	1,070	1,042
Kansas	551	646	609	680	682	875	770	649	643	633
Kentucky	874	895	886	930	1,206	1,355	1,596	1,546	1,424	1,448
Louisiana	1,564	1,383	1,924	1,823	1,990	1,956	2,054	2,591	2,653	2,649
Maine	190	179	185	270	250	199	76	76	53	0
Maryland	286	261	256	321	399	346	273	311	315	322
Massachusetts	852	758	767	817	815	935	811	942	955	932
Michigan	1,437	1,163	1,250	1,040	1,027	1,216	992	908	1,027	758
Minnesota	1,185	1,213	1,354	1,691	2,021	2,520	2,305	2,838	2,527	2,121
Mississippi	491	617	531	621	658	727	767	799	777	892
Missouri	931	995	901	1,092	1,117	1,261	1,471	1,449	1,829	1,563
Montana	205	180	191	241	246	220	227	219	240	234
Nebraska	434	369	433	568	439	423	453	444	425	365
Nevada	64	56	87	69	48	90	66	72	88	72
New Hampshire	106	62	89	124	45	118	125	126	137	140
New Jersey	1,504	1,278	1,343	1,448	1,616	1,766	1,670	1,598	1,793	1,597
New Mexico	234	242	209	136	209	161	189	161	209	226
New York	3,413	2,950	2,937	3,441	4,123	3,990	4,791	5,573	5,342	4,920
North Carolina	608	569	576	596	627	730	966	1,037	1,114	832
North Dakota	56	235	220	20	108	159	147	177	142	87
Ohio	1,672	1,640	1,856	2,176	2,498	2,591	2,361	2,552	2,586	2,474
Oklahoma	825	689	804	893	955	1,061	1,110	1,178	1,083	1,225
Oregon	390	310	66	0	94	0	0	0	110	42
Pennsylvania	2,249	1,918	1,866	2,136	2,471	2,824	2,807	2,785	2,869	2,433
Rhode Island	114	0	0	0	291	0	0	0	0	0
South Carolina	600	544	565	727	843	892	945	885	938	865
South Dakota	14	20	26	24	68	77	59	70	67	63
Tennessee	961	1,025	1,187	1,378	1,410	1,620	1,243	1,584	1,498	1,350
Texas	4,294	4,113	4,471	4,408	4,776	5,185	5,258	5,384	5,521	5,378
Utah	281	289	328	444	330	359	426	375	425	380
Vermont	114	51	80	88	105	90	104	80	99	84
Virginia	1,477	1,350	1,313	1,426	1,461	1,728	1,777	1,881	1,825	1,865
Washington	1,175	1,116	828	722	820	698	694	809	685	701
West Virginia	462	481	517	575	550	608	641	633	634	608
Wisconsin	222	197	218	279	232	286	308	322	254	260
Wyoming	88	112	126	63	177	54	24	0	24	40
American Samoa	7	7	7	15	15	15	15	10	0	27
Guam	0	0	0	0	0	0	0	0	0	0
Puerto Rico	1,518	1,302	693	842	1,159	1,225	1,385	1,391	1,893	2,182
Virgin Islands	0	0	22	22	13	30	34	35	13	30

[1] National and regional totals exclude American Samoa, Guam, Puerto Rico, and the Virgin Islands.

Table 7
ANNUAL ADMISSIONS TO LPN/LVN PROGRAMS, BY NLN REGION
AND PRIMARY SOURCE OF FINANCIAL SUPPORT: 1985-86 TO 1994-95

NLN REGION BY TYPE OF FINANCIAL SUPPORT [1]	NUMBER OF ANNUAL ADMISSIONS									
	1985-86	1986-87	1987-88	1988-89	1989-90	1990-91	1991-92	1992-93	1993-94	1994-95
All Regions	**44,477**	**42,452**	**43,774**	**47,602**	**52,969**	**56,176**	**58,245**	**60,749**	**60,632**	**57,906**
Public	41,056	39,103	40,116	43,678	48,729	50,998	53,379	55,551	55,187	51,555
Private	3,421	3,349	3,658	3,924	4,240	5,178	4,866	5,198	5,445	6,351
North Atlantic	9,332	7,789	7,985	8,972	10,558	10,653	11,156	11,896	11,986	10,969
Public	7,998	6,651	6,801	7,585	8,917	8,561	9,258	9,843	9,751	8,485
Private	1,334	1,138	1,184	1,387	1,641	2,092	1,898	2,053	2,235	2,484
Midwest	9,556	10,145	10,256	11,332	12,802	13,857	13,534	14,115	14,580	13,145
Public	9,271	9,692	10,000	10,857	12,350	13,335	12,936	13,731	13,756	12,425
Private	285	453	256	475	452	522	598	384	824	720
South	18,404	17,779	19,073	21,087	22,743	25,049	26,365	27,544	27,956	27,400
Public	17,708	17,095	18,239	20,065	21,413	23,405	24,698	25,825	25,964	25,374
Private	696	684	834	1,022	1,330	1,644	1,667	1,719	1,992	2,026
West	7,185	6,739	6,460	6,211	6,866	6,617	7,190	7,194	6,110	6,392
Public	6,079	5,665	5,076	5,171	6,049	5,697	6,487	6,152	5,716	5,271
Private	1,106	1,074	1,384	1,040	817	920	703	1,042	394	1,121

[1] Excludes American Samoa, Guam, Puerto Rico, and the Virgin Islands.

145

Table 8
ANNUAL ADMISSIONS TO LPN/LVN PROGRAMS, BY NLN REGION
AND TYPE OF ADMINISTRATIVE CONTROL: 1985-86 TO 1994-95

NLN REGION BY TYPE OF ADMINISTRATIVE CONTROL [1]	NUMBER OF ANNUAL ADMISSIONS									
	1985-86	1986-87	1987-88	1988-89	1989-90	1990-91	1991-92	1992-93	1993-94	1994-95
All Regions	**44,477**	**42,452**	**43,774**	**47,602**	**52,969**	**56,176**	**58,245**	**60,749**	**60,632**	**57,906**
Technical or vocational school	25,156	23,722	25,251	27,528	30,101	32,045	34,291	36,079	34,866	32,977
Junior or community college	12,941	13,385	13,620	13,895	16,172	17,453	17,124	17,370	18,809	17,503
Secondary school	3,379	2,700	2,330	3,127	3,322	3,170	3,338	3,830	3,663	3,790
Hospital	1,178	1,000	1,230	1,690	1,702	1,590	1,501	1,637	1,563	1,689
Government agency	1,211	1,237	1,056	937	1,072	1,080	1,038	946	924	865
Senior college or university	297	142	137	195	231	450	505	467	352	481
Independent agency	315	266	150	230	369	388	448	420	455	601
North Atlantic	9,332	7,789	7,985	8,972	10,558	10,653	11,156	11,896	11,986	10,969
Technical or vocational school	5,976	5,172	5,773	5,957	7,091	7,421	8,333	8,454	8,347	7,927
Junior or community college	1,174	882	792	873	1,256	1,176	885	1,070	1,343	1,077
Secondary school	1,487	1,199	858	1,251	1,362	1,028	862	1,302	1,440	875
Hospital	525	397	482	741	695	721	717	747	649	737
Government agency	83	128	80	82	88	95	74	92	74	39
Senior college or university	0	0	0	68	66	212	255	209	111	100
Independent agency	87	11	0	0	0	0	30	22	22	214
Midwest	9,556	10,145	10,256	11,332	12,802	13,857	13,534	14,115	14,580	13,145
Technical or vocational school	5,368	5,585	5,589	6,267	7,419	8,505	7,860	8,768	8,923	7,733
Junior or community college	3,575	3,698	4,005	4,066	4,433	4,615	4,737	4,417	4,898	4,292
Secondary school	472	452	415	689	417	303	723	717	540	908
Hospital	69	89	89	109	93	82	94	54	32	99
Government agency	0	258	107	108	275	252	0	0	54	0
Senior college or university	39	42	25	0	40	40	40	80	40	113
Independent agency	33	21	26	93	125	60	80	119	93	0
South	18,404	17,779	19,073	21,087	22,743	25,049	26,365	27,544	27,956	27,400
Technical or vocational school	11,026	10,722	11,340	12,852	13,240	13,525	14,828	15,234	15,570	14,904
Junior or community college	4,712	5,025	5,612	5,923	6,834	8,638	8,459	9,043	9,337	9,002
Secondary school	795	587	553	683	1,043	1,207	1,142	1,256	1,042	1,347
Hospital	584	514	659	840	854	787	690	776	802	823
Government agency	1,128	851	837	709	657	691	920	818	780	794
Senior college or university	56	30	29	40	40	70	121	138	120	143
Independent agency	103	50	43	40	75	131	205	279	305	387
West	7,185	6,739	6,460	6,211	6,866	6,617	7,190	7,194	6,110	6,392
Technical or vocational school	2,786	2,243	2,549	2,452	2,351	2,594	3,270	3,623	2,026	2,413
Junior or community college	3,480	3,780	3,211	3,033	3,649	3,024	3,043	2,840	3,231	3,132
Secondary school	625	462	504	504	500	632	611	555	641	660
Hospital	0	0	0	0	60	0	0	60	80	30
Government agency	0	0	32	38	52	42	44	36	16	32
Senior college or university	202	70	83	87	85	128	89	80	81	125
Independent agency	92	184	81	97	169	197	133	0	35	0

[1] Excludes American Samoa, Guam, Puerto Rico, and the Virgin Islands.

146

Table 9
FALL ADMISSIONS TO LPN/LVN PROGRAMS
WITH PERCENTAGE CHANGE FROM PREVIOUS YEAR:
1980 TO 1995

YEAR[1]	FALL ADMISSIONS	
	Number[2]	Percent Change
1980	37,044	+2.4
1981	38,236	+3.2
1982	39,560	+3.4
1983	37,788	-4.5
1984	33,351	-11.7
1985	29,067	-12.8
1986	27,816	-4.3
1987	28,274	+1.7
1988	30,746	+8.7
1989	31,905	+3.8
1990	33,232	+4.2
1991	36,503	+9.0
1992	36,228	-0.7
1993	37,932	+4.7
1994	36,842	-2.9
1995	34,733	-5.7

[1] Time period is August 1 through December 31.
[2] Excludes American Samoa, Guam, Puerto Rico, and the Virgin Islands.

Table 10
FALL ADMISSIONS TO LPN/LVN PROGRAMS, BY NLN REGION AND STATE: 1986 TO 1995

NLN REGION AND STATE	NUMBER OF FALL ADMISSIONS									
	1986	1987	1988	1989	1990	1991	1992	1993	1994	1995
United States[1]	**27,816**	**28,274**	**30,746**	**31,905**	**33,232**	**36,503**	**36,228**	**37,932**	**36,842**	**34,733**
North Atlantic	6,423	5,572	6,680	7,090	7,698	8,729	8,460	8,610	8,187	7,765
Midwest	6,466	7,125	7,620	8,192	8,826	9,539	8,837	9,422	9,232	8,589
South	11,477	11,944	12,616	12,745	13,401	14,693	15,073	16,305	15,213	15,001
West	3,450	3,633	3,830	3,878	3,307	3,542	3,858	3,595	4,210	3,378
Alabama	728	675	822	904	1,240	1,222	1,106	1,869	1,232	1,131
Alaska	0	0	0	0	0	0	0	0	0	0
Arizona	205	146	240	234	226	239	246	336	292	191
Arkansas	564	607	632	578	654	675	592	607	685	642
California	1,780	1,812	1,968	2,137	1,482	1,810	1,969	1,671	2,161	1,486
Colorado	236	322	346	271	336	329	404	235	349	321
Connecticut	132	32	194	61	109	450	317	145	254	412
Delaware	75	80	98	63	43	105	79	78	100	112
District of Columbia	196	146	191	124	120	98	40	61	74	172
Florida	1,119	1,193	1,328	1,255	1,512	1,528	1,411	1,531	1,748	1,759
Georgia	897	749	713	680	697	923	865	1,058	860	1,021
Hawaii	107	83	74	109	40	52	109	78	143	231
Idaho	73	71	101	107	117	117	124	138	100	89
Illinois	1,117	1,242	1,094	1,213	1,306	1,462	1,330	1,525	1,301	1,234
Indiana	596	642	823	948	1,050	1,202	959	1,265	1,133	1,027
Iowa	444	478	525	583	716	783	759	641	679	680
Kansas	434	377	376	445	423	568	506	435	486	509
Kentucky	585	469	678	614	551	760	870	793	740	751
Louisiana	593	809	625	925	552	822	1,347	1,167	900	1,026
Maine	198	124	202	210	200	171	51	51	45	0
Maryland	208	171	231	318	300	323	239	279	204	255
Massachusetts	730	759	862	824	793	783	764	960	923	947
Michigan	793	765	810	551	854	851	720	685	594	597
Minnesota	804	1,068	1,160	1,276	1,212	1,480	1,296	1,249	1,457	1,465
Mississippi	372	270	478	472	555	538	623	589	654	850
Missouri	720	724	724	874	939	992	1,068	1,155	1,257	1,028
Montana	106	167	158	153	139	137	142	157	138	131
Nebraska	240	245	359	351	266	280	261	362	331	212
Nevada	60	46	31	21	86	86	72	48	40	40
New Hampshire	102	56	89	94	103	59	55	109	110	118
New Jersey	981	984	1,095	1,257	1,219	1,412	1,297	1,338	1,036	916
New Mexico	134	145	197	150	163	159	165	157	219	172
New York	2,673	2,273	2,792	3,175	3,343	3,896	4,345	4,303	4,012	3,758
North Carolina	526	451	550	540	516	630	636	719	747	639
North Dakota	68	26	76	18	58	32	67	89	124	64
Ohio	1,098	1,369	1,478	1,721	1,732	1,620	1,581	1,717	1,607	1,539
Oklahoma	621	590	658	785	910	969	950	945	792	730
Oregon	67	101	66	0	0	0	0	0	90	24
Pennsylvania	1,285	1,038	1,093	1,178	1,370	1,649	1,412	1,464	1,549	1,228
Rhode Island	0	0	0	0	308	0	0	0	0	0
South Carolina	487	499	504	511	602	655	627	670	562	558
South Dakota	20	24	23	67	73	64	66	105	63	31
Tennessee	596	610	706	696	768	662	700	895	726	720
Texas	2,608	3,227	2,940	2,675	2,825	2,944	2,966	3,289	3,378	2,942
Utah	122	189	180	165	160	219	262	225	245	171
Vermont	51	80	64	104	90	106	100	101	84	102
Virginia	1,230	1,223	1,330	1,353	1,357	1,569	1,602	1,519	1,559	1,610
Washington	496	479	388	472	480	368	365	550	433	482
West Virginia	343	401	421	439	362	473	539	375	426	367
Wisconsin	132	165	172	145	197	205	224	194	200	203
Wyoming	64	72	81	59	78	26	0	0	0	40
American Samoa	7	7	7	8	15	15	15	0	0	0
Guam	0	0	0	0	0	0	0	0	0	0
Puerto Rico	911	832	459	528	667	394	811	832	769	919
Virgin Islands	0	0	13	13	0	34	21	0	0	42

[1] National and regional totals exclude American Samoa, Guam, Puerto Rico, and the Virgin Islands.

Table 11
FALL ADMISSIONS TO LPN/LVN PROGRAMS
BY NLN REGION AND PRIMARY SOURCE OF FINANCIAL SUPPORT: 1986 TO 1995

NLN REGION BY TYPE OF FINANCIAL SUPPORT[1]	NUMBER OF FALL ADMISSIONS									
	1986	1987	1988	1989	1990	1991	1992	1993	1994	1995
All Regions	**27,816**	**28,274**	**30,746**	**31,905**	**33,232**	**36,503**	**36,228**	**37,932**	**36,842**	**34,733**
Public	25,766	25,890	27,993	29,469	30,633	33,562	33,292	34,938	33,639	31,526
Private	2,050	2,384	2,753	2,436	2,599	2,941	2,936	2,994	3,203	3,207
North Atlantic	6,423	5,572	6,680	7,090	7,698	8,729	8,460	8,610	8,187	7,765
Public	5,380	4,592	5,416	5,915	6,364	7,140	6,859	7,095	6,578	6,095
Private	1,043	980	1,264	1,175	1,334	1,589	1,601	1,515	1,609	1,670
Midwest	6,466	7,125	7,620	8,192	8,826	9,539	8,837	9,422	9,232	8,589
Public	6,266	6,847	7,440	7,856	8,436	9,174	8,518	9,202	8,776	8,278
Private	200	278	180	336	390	365	319	220	456	311
South	11,477	11,944	12,616	12,745	13,401	14,693	15,073	16,305	15,213	15,001
Public	11,111	11,343	11,890	12,124	12,627	13,856	14,208	15,302	14,317	14,025
Private	366	601	726	621	774	837	865	1,003	896	976
West	3,450	3,633	3,830	3,878	3,307	3,542	3,858	3,595	4,210	3,378
Public	3,009	3,108	3,247	3,574	3,206	3,392	3,707	3,339	3,968	3,128
Private	441	525	583	304	101	150	151	256	242	250

[1] Excludes American Samoa, Guam, Puerto Rico, and the Virgin Islands.

149

Table 12
FALL ADMISSIONS TO LPN/LVN PROGRAMS, BY NLN REGION
AND TYPE OF ADMINISTRATIVE CONTROL: 1986 TO 1995

NLN REGION BY TYPE OF ADMINISTRATIVE CONTROL [1]	NUMBER OF FALL ADMISSIONS									
	1986	1987	1988	1989	1990	1991	1992	1993	1994	1995
All Regions	**27,816**	**28,274**	**30,746**	**31,905**	**33,232**	**36,503**	**36,228**	**37,932**	**36,842**	**34,733**
Technical or vocational school	15,882	15,655	17,469	18,141	18,407	21,130	21,395	21,395	20,436	19,125
Junior or community college	7,904	8,582	9,681	9,553	10,632	11,528	10,913	11,974	11,975	11,321
Secondary school	2,335	2,166	1,749	2,336	2,147	1,987	2,240	2,467	2,385	2,564
Hospital	758	794	1,191	1,115	1,160	1,061	975	1,126	1,002	819
Government agency	611	850	396	416	506	277	83	326	518	278
Senior college or university	150	71	145	185	199	363	406	409	281	378
Independent agency	176	156	115	159	181	157	216	235	245	248
North Atlantic	6,423	5,572	6,680	7,090	7,698	8,729	8,460	8,610	8,187	7,765
Technical or vocational school	4,119	3,458	4,753	4,785	5,272	6,169	6,370	6,071	5,412	5,639
Junior or community college	726	641	577	779	1,019	1,023	705	859	1,103	866
Secondary school	1,082	993	655	791	637	675	545	861	962	600
Hospital	358	314	615	582	600	531	494	517	522	382
Government agency	53	152	80	88	103	96	68	99	87	39
Senior college or university	0	0	0	65	67	235	248	182	80	110
Independent agency	85	14	0	0	0	0	30	21	21	129
Midwest	6,466	7,125	7,620	8,192	8,826	9,539	8,837	9,422	9,232	8,589
Technical or vocational college	3,675	4,153	4,381	4,873	5,148	5,711	5,020	5,392	5,534	4,831
Junior or community college	2,382	2,521	2,796	2,750	3,176	3,351	3,259	3,391	3,279	2,998
Secondary school	351	342	258	395	257	232	461	491	302	622
Hospital	22	22	30	27	27	70	55	31	34	22
Government agency	0	87	65	70	136	135	0	0	0	0
Senior college or university	36	0	50	29	40	0	0	40	38	116
Independent agency	0	0	40	48	42	40	42	77	45	0
South	11,477	11,944	12,616	12,745	13,401	14,693	15,073	16,305	15,213	15,001
Technical or vocational school	6,737	6,552	6,874	7,265	7,080	7,970	8,680	8,423	7,887	7,641
Junior or community college	3,034	3,644	4,349	4,096	4,580	5,425	4,986	5,986	5,507	5,493
Secondary school	644	598	528	567	833	741	759	878	711	962
Hospital	378	458	546	506	533	460	426	518	446	415
Government agency	558	611	228	232	246	28	15	227	415	239
Senior college or university	60	29	40	40	40	36	108	136	93	132
Independent agency	66	52	51	39	89	33	99	137	154	119
West	3,450	3,633	3,830	3,878	3,307	3,542	3,858	3,595	4,210	3,378
Technical or vocational school	1,351	1,492	1,461	1,218	907	1,280	1,325	1,509	1,603	1,014
Junior or community college	1,762	1,776	1,959	1,928	1,857	1,729	1,963	1,738	2,086	1,964
Secondary school	258	233	308	583	420	339	475	237	410	380
Hospital	0	0	0	0	0	0	0	60	0	0
Government agency	0	0	23	26	21	18	0	0	16	0
Senior college or university	54	42	55	51	52	92	50	51	70	20
Independent agency	25	90	24	72	50	84	45	0	25	0

[1] Excludes American Samoa, Guam, Puerto Rico, and the Virgin Islands.

150

Table 13
ENROLLMENTS IN LPN/LVN PROGRAMS
WITH PERCENTAGE CHANGE FROM PREVIOUS YEAR: 1976 TO 1995

YEAR	ENROLLMENTS	
	Number[1]	Percent Change
1976	58,423	- 0.1
1977	56,943	- 2.5
1978	54,543	- 4.2
1979	52,202	- 4.3
1980	52,565	+ 0.7
1981	55,024	+ 4.7
1982	57,367	+ 4.2
1983	55,446	- 3.4
1984	48,840	-11.9
1985	39,345	-19.4
1986	38,510	- 2.1
1987	40,035	+ 4.0
1988	42,808	+ 6.9
1989	46,720	+ 9.1
1990	52,749	+12.9
1991	56,762	+ 7.1
1992	59,095	+ 4.1
1993	61,007	+ 3.2
1994	59,428	- 2.6
1995	56,028	- 5.7

[1] Excludes American Samoa, Guam, Puerto Rico, and the Virgin Islands.

Table 14
ENROLLMENTS IN LPN/LVN PROGRAMS, BY NLN REGION AND STATE: 1986 TO 1995

NLN REGION AND STATE	NUMBER OF ENROLLMENTS									
	1986	1987	1988	1989	1990	1991	1992	1993	1994	1995
United States[1]	**38,510**	**40,035**	**42,808**	**46,720**	**52,749**	**56,762**	**59,095**	**61,007**	**59,428**	**56,028**
North Atlantic	8,125	7,731	8,615	9,595	11,215	12,168	12,355	12,944	12,445	10,877
Midwest	8,629	9,787	10,583	11,370	12,902	13,945	13,998	14,846	14,629	13,305
South	15,562	16,241	17,674	19,242	21,678	23,925	25,620	25,852	25,765	25,503
West	6,194	6,276	5,936	6,513	6,954	6,724	7,122	7,365	6,589	6,343
Alabama	1,010	1,131	1,254	1,578	2,252	2,432	3,060	2,601	2,846	2,921
Alaska	0	0	0	0	0	0	0	0	0	0
Arizona	280	343	283	360	408	395	322	484	315	333
Arkansas	624	894	699	837	782	905	952	892	847	922
California	3,431	3,087	3,328	4,013	3,886	4,087	4,477	4,496	3,609	3,593
Colorado	282	504	368	419	409	400	561	386	519	412
Connecticut	249	242	207	294	383	465	390	398	493	457
Delaware	60	90	86	149	202	114	130	128	251	135
District of Columbia	244	148	202	110	236	199	200	178	215	226
Florida	1,658	1,924	2,070	2,299	2,690	3,026	3,057	2,960	3,132	3,214
Georgia	1,170	1,226	1,318	1,380	1,720	1,965	2,154	2,229	2,275	2,258
Hawaii	126	110	109	112	167	106	101	73	197	228
Idaho	107	97	116	117	131	139	142	155	149	148
Illinois	1,335	1,594	1,570	1,697	2,066	2,052	1,843	1,896	2,056	2,024
Indiana	803	936	1,118	1,233	1,364	1,886	1,512	2,079	1,959	1,820
Iowa	626	925	877	853	1,095	1,079	1,077	1,013	1,193	1,244
Kansas	619	543	571	610	707	741	708	622	589	605
Kentucky	701	771	781	842	1,052	1,327	1,475	1,394	1,280	1,180
Louisiana	1,132	1,193	1,270	1,585	1,498	1,582	1,887	2,031	2,030	1,955
Maine	184	168	213	254	235	164	48	48	45	0
Maryland	308	247	299	397	424	428	380	373	375	377
Massachusetts	746	781	875	813	800	879	835	1,003	1,008	966
Michigan	1,256	1,148	1,250	1,034	1,371	1,149	1,073	992	1,170	916
Minnesota	1,004	1,145	1,429	1,768	2,021	2,528	3,029	3,060	2,648	2,216
Mississippi	523	520	400	566	653	609	719	728	747	891
Missouri	894	869	977	1,086	1,097	1,220	1,353	1,509	1,656	1,435
Montana	166	161	230	229	257	255	255	273	254	258
Nebraska	388	462	476	465	330	414	406	424	356	314
Nevada	60	52	42	73	86	83	72	47	75	70
New Hampshire	103	102	122	141	143	165	178	165	184	194
New Jersey	1,115	1,393	1,561	1,869	1,720	1,955	1,870	2,116	1,970	1,858
New Mexico	248	260	228	137	225	152	165	157	228	165
New York	3,395	3,027	3,329	3,717	4,646	5,259	5,759	6,081	5,447	4,641
North Carolina	560	504	563	581	634	752	917	1,113	1,048	824
North Dakota	82	166	165	21	172	250	314	251	246	119
Ohio	1,463	1,777	1,925	2,316	2,392	2,347	2,353	2,526	2,399	2,258
Oklahoma	730	712	837	890	1,039	1,122	1,097	1,091	1,072	1,167
Oregon	240	256	56	0	94	0	0	0	110	47
Pennsylvania	1,948	1,698	1,938	2,148	2,438	2,867	2,849	2,732	2,737	2,306
Rhode Island	0	0	0	0	304	0	0	0	0	0
South Carolina	573	556	627	755	789	897	878	918	922	778
South Dakota	20	24	26	66	73	60	64	67	63	63
Tennessee	763	893	1,045	1,118	1,200	1,246	1,172	1,398	1,213	1,197
Texas	3,610	3,477	4,273	4,070	4,361	4,923	5,063	5,162	5,026	4,902
Utah	259	279	335	376	318	359	357	370	419	369
Vermont	81	82	82	100	108	101	96	95	95	94
Virginia	1,766	1,776	1,763	1,835	2,056	2,157	2,273	2,355	2,397	2,374
Washington	915	1,032	701	605	795	700	653	924	690	681
West Virginia	434	417	475	509	528	554	536	607	555	543
Wisconsin	139	198	199	221	214	219	266	407	294	291
Wyoming	80	95	140	72	178	48	17	0	24	39
American Samoa	14	14	14	15	8	8	8	12	0	19
Guam	0	0	0	0	0	0	0	0	0	0
Puerto Rico	1,801	1,607	1,043	1,341	1,268	1,405	1,559	1,413	2,462	2,718
Virgin Islands	0	0	13	13	10	59	28	25	13	69

[1] National and regional totals exclude American Samoa, Guam, Puerto Rico, and the Virgin Islands.

Table 15
ENROLLMENTS IN LPN/LVN PROGRAMS
BY NLN REGION AND PRIMARY SOURCE OF FINANCIAL SUPPORT: 1986 TO 1995

NLN REGION BY TYPE OF FINANCIAL SUPPORT [1]	NUMBER OF ENROLLMENTS									
	1986	1987	1988	1989	1990	1991	1992	1993	1994	1995
All Regions	**38,510**	**40,035**	**42,808**	**46,720**	**52,749**	**56,762**	**59,095**	**61,007**	**59,428**	**56,028**
Public	35,785	37,133	39,249	43,132	48,649	51,510	54,330	56,120	54,136	50,365
Private	2,725	2,902	3,559	3,588	4,100	5,252	4,765	4,887	5,292	5,663
North Atlantic	8,125	7,731	8,615	9,595	11,215	12,168	12,355	12,944	12,445	10,877
Public	7,046	6,659	7,214	8,210	9,517	9,877	10,180	10,773	10,176	8,630
Private	1,079	1,072	1,401	1,385	1,698	2,291	2,175	2,171	2,269	2,247
Midwest	8,629	9,787	10,583	11,370	12,902	13,945	13,998	14,846	14,629	13,305
Public	8,378	9,386	10,289	10,974	12,520	13,469	13,594	14,461	13,910	12,717
Private	251	401	294	396	382	476	404	385	719	588
South	15,562	16,241	17,674	19,242	21,678	23,925	25,620	25,852	25,765	25,503
Public	15,037	15,613	16,810	18,266	20,443	22,345	24,008	24,205	23,931	23,594
Private	525	628	864	976	1,235	1,580	1,612	1,647	1,834	1,909
West	6,194	6,276	5,936	6,513	6,954	6,724	7,122	7,365	6,589	6,343
Public	5,324	5,475	4,936	5,682	6,169	5,819	6,548	6,681	6,119	5,424
Private	870	801	1,000	831	785	905	574	684	470	919

[1] Excludes American Samoa, Guam, Puerto Rico, and the Virgin Islands.

Table 16
ENROLLMENTS IN LPN/LVN PROGRAMS, BY NLN REGION AND ADMINISTRATIVE CONTROL: 1986 TO 1995

NLN REGION BY TYPE OF ADMINISTRATIVE CONTROL [1]	NUMBER OF ENROLLMENTS									
	1986	1987	1988	1989	1990	1991	1992	1993	1994	1995
All Regions	**38,510**	**40,035**	**42,808**	**46,720**	**52,749**	**56,762**	**59,095**	**61,007**	**59,428**	**56,028**
Technical or vocational school	21,405	21,931	24,047	26,501	29,672	32,863	35,167	35,691	33,714	31,534
Junior or community college	11,347	12,979	13,297	13,719	16,421	17,313	16,850	17,688	18,272	17,199
Secondary school	3,391	3,134	2,673	3,675	3,599	3,288	3,726	4,115	4,114	4,075
Hospital	891	933	1,396	1,548	1,601	1,577	1,545	1,577	1,562	1,444
Government agency	940	700	1,061	840	898	1,069	950	932	1,024	803
Senior college or university	298	109	147	199	237	452	523	582	319	493
Independent agency	238	249	187	238	321	200	334	422	423	480
North Atlantic	8,125	7,731	8,615	9,595	11,215	12,168	12,355	12,944	12,445	10,877
Technical or vocational school	5,204	5,043	6,068	6,421	7,540	8,724	9,365	9,048	8,539	7,951
Junior or community college	890	782	804	999	1,403	1,249	913	1,339	1,429	1,162
Secondary school	1,518	1,345	1,010	1,352	1,400	1,102	979	1,366	1,448	833
Hospital	372	394	655	676	707	764	757	799	752	635
Government agency	59	153	78	83	101	110	64	95	179	38
Senior college or university	0	0	0	64	64	219	255	277	78	105
Independent agency	82	14	0	0	0	0	22	20	20	153
Midwest	8,629	9,787	10,583	11,370	12,902	13,945	13,998	14,846	14,629	13,305
Technical or vocational college	4,837	5,245	5,719	6,550	7,353	8,517	8,496	9,320	8,786	7,717
Junior or community college	3,273	3,738	4,181	3,850	4,790	4,663	4,598	4,614	5,100	4,501
Secondary school	416	514	404	689	346	342	687	669	534	897
Hospital	59	68	95	92	78	72	73	64	34	57
Government agency	0	190	96	104	213	225	0	0	57	0
Senior college or university	35	18	34	29	61	62	69	68	38	133
Independent agency	9	14	54	56	61	64	75	111	80	0
South	15,562	16,241	17,674	19,242	21,678	23,925	25,620	25,852	25,765	25,503
Technical or vocational school	9,031	9,634	10,085	11,382	12,485	12,974	14,210	13,970	14,119	13,640
Junior or community college	4,084	4,833	5,260	5,582	6,487	8,180	8,171	8,426	8,363	8,316
Secondary school	939	882	739	789	1,221	1,145	1,328	1,476	1,351	1,583
Hospital	460	471	646	780	766	741	715	714	746	724
Government agency	881	357	856	630	575	710	864	813	772	765
Senior college or university	84	28	38	40	40	59	125	162	118	148
Independent agency	83	36	50	39	104	116	207	291	296	327
West	6,194	6,276	5,936	6,513	6,954	6,724	7,122	7,365	6,589	6,343
Technical or vocational school	2,333	2,009	2,175	2,148	2,294	2,648	3,096	3,353	2,270	2,226
Junior or community college	3,100	3,626	3,052	3,288	3,741	3,221	3,168	3,309	3,380	3,220
Secondary school	518	393	520	845	632	699	732	604	781	762
Hospital	0	0	0	0	50	0	0	0	30	28
Government agency	0	0	31	23	9	24	22	24	16	0
Senior college or university	179	63	75	66	72	112	74	75	85	107
Independent agency	64	185	83	143	156	20	30	0	27	0

[1] Excludes American Samoa, Guam, Puerto Rico, and the Virgin Islands.

Table 17
GRADUATIONS FROM LPN/LVN PROGRAMS WITH PERCENTAGE CHANGE FROM PREVIOUS YEAR: 1975-76 TO 1994-95

YEAR[1]	GRADUATIONS [2]		YEAR[1]	GRADUATIONS [2]	
	Number	Percent Change		Number	Percent Change
1975-76	47,145	+ 3.9	1985-86	29,599	-19.9
1976-77	46,614	- 1.1	1986-87	27,285	- 7.8
1977-78	45,350	- 2.7	1987-88	26,912	- 1.4
1978-79	44,235	- 2.5	1988-89	30,368	+12.8
1979-80	41,892	- 5.3	1989-90	35,417	+16.6
1980-81	41,002	- 2.1	1990-91	38,100	+ 7.0
1981-82	43,299	+ 5.6	1991-92	41,951	+10.1
1982-83	45,174	+ 4.3	1992-93	44,822	+ 6.8
1983-84	44,654	- 2.5	1993-94	45,083	+ 0.6
1984-85	36,955	-17.2	1994-95	44,234	- 1.9

[1] Time period is September 1 through August 31 for academic years 1973-74 through 1981-82, and August 1 through July 31 for subsequent years.
[2] Excludes American Samoa, Guam, Puerto Rico, and the Virgin Islands.

Table 18
GRADUATIONS FROM LPN/LVN PROGRAMS, BY NLN REGION AND STATE: 1985-86 TO 1994-95

NLN REGION AND STATE	NUMBER OF GRADUATIONS									
	1985-86	1986-87	1987-88	1988-89	1989-90	1990-91	1991-92	1992-93	1993-94	1994-95
United States[1]	**29,599**	**27,285**	**26,912**	**30,368**	**35,417**	**38,100**	**41,951**	**44,822**	**45,083**	**44,234**
North Atlantic	6,168	5,207	4,856	5,595	6,493	7,175	7,659	8,676	9,058	8,616
Midwest	7,085	6,619	6,839	7,536	9,116	9,651	10,603	11,167	11,308	10,883
South	11,703	10,879	10,693	12,236	14,256	15,708	17,476	18,484	18,663	18,723
West	4,643	4,580	4,524	5,001	5,552	5,566	6,213	6,495	6,054	6,012
Alabama	812	783	749	830	1,190	1,214	1,717	1,852	1,644	1,718
Alaska	0	0	0	0	0	0	0	0	0	0
Arizona	243	316	275	301	340	419	450	538	543	472
Arkansas	504	625	540	606	602	695	793	751	755	665
California	2,343	2,207	2,039	2,265	2,462	2,449	2,847	3,111	2,546	2,735
Colorado	269	260	323	395	434	501	483	583	602	579
Connecticut	256	257	246	217	342	362	119	316	377	395
Delaware	64	44	55	59	62	60	81	69	108	79
District of Columbia	44	61	42	54	62	79	48	27	127	236
Florida	1,512	1,374	1,428	1,522	2,018	2,143	2,480	2,446	2,529	2,503
Georgia	923	883	794	933	942	1,015	1,084	1,191	1,308	1,286
Hawaii	97	63	71	77	91	131	116	111	136	189
Idaho	74	90	90	107	107	113	130	129	112	142
Illinois	1,296	1,030	1,100	1,176	1,376	1,553	1,506	1,718	1,577	1,563
Indiana	674	669	699	730	893	949	1,187	1,376	1,419	1,380
Iowa	397	489	581	632	809	893	966	1,052	1,020	977
Kansas	419	469	531	510	656	705	692	646	638	598
Kentucky	545	596	554	582	682	852	1,131	1,207	917	1,057
Louisiana	798	763	699	841	885	1,057	991	1,110	1,383	1,271
Maine	146	152	131	182	204	198	149	134	49	34
Maryland	204	175	178	211	276	246	291	288	290	331
Massachusetts	590	541	550	629	714	677	717	702	744	762
Michigan	1,013	955	767	787	1,031	956	1,214	1,052	1,068	1,027
Minnesota	715	718	752	914	1,110	1,174	1,452	1,409	1,276	1,296
Mississippi	360	418	324	343	408	500	541	551	599	699
Missouri	819	644	666	726	850	1,059	1,111	1,121	1,386	1,273
Montana	106	100	121	128	161	149	151	147	140	134
Nebraska	255	227	290	353	336	319	312	314	328	315
Nevada	45	43	56	49	63	79	73	88	73	99
New Hampshire	80	56	74	32	87	82	92	104	99	108
New Jersey	1,052	814	740	830	871	1,081	1,228	1,150	1,205	1,268
New Mexico	197	152	135	130	142	155	170	177	207	236
New York	2,059	1,844	1,630	1,972	2,345	2,535	2,972	3,712	3,884	3,254
North Carolina	463	329	314	367	430	469	610	605	721	655
North Dakota	42	44	78	38	80	55	104	140	164	143
Ohio	1,300	1,215	1,227	1,443	1,723	1,681	1,773	1,936	2,075	1,996
Oklahoma	594	489	539	693	766	812	934	968	878	887
Oregon	315	265	309	289	350	309	369	232	281	201
Pennsylvania	1,709	1,336	1,282	1,506	1,678	1,970	2,127	2,326	2,325	2,333
Rhode Island	79	45	48	48	59	52	51	51	63	63
South Carolina	362	321	317	359	449	431	457	542	489	546
South Dakota	13	17	19	21	52	61	50	59	62	58
Tennessee	597	655	702	781	964	1,089	935	1,001	1,083	949
Texas	2,750	2,397	2,437	2,998	3,367	3,817	4,090	4,376	4,384	4,503
Utah	237	233	266	328	341	272	364	353	386	401
Vermont	89	57	58	66	69	79	75	85	77	84
Virginia	840	751	778	778	853	906	928	1,072	1,159	1,132
Washington	658	784	765	830	946	876	931	926	951	726
West Virginia	439	320	340	392	424	462	494	524	524	521
Wisconsin	142	142	129	206	200	246	236	344	295	257
Wyoming	59	67	74	102	115	113	129	100	77	98
American Samoa	8	8	8	8	8	8	8	9	0	0
Guam	0	0	0	0	0	0	0	0	0	0
Puerto Rico	1,086	931	501	511	665	868	801	734	1,157	1,314
Virgin Islands	0	0	15	15	8	11	28	9	7	20

[1] National and regional totals exclude American Samoa, Guam, Puerto Rico, and the Virgin Islands.

Table 19
GRADUATIONS FROM LPN/LVN PROGRAMS,
BY NLN REGION AND PRIMARY SOURCE OF FINANCIAL SUPPORT: 1985-86 TO 1994-95

NLN REGION BY TYPE OF FINANCIAL SUPPORT [1]	NUMBER OF GRADUATIONS									
	1985-86	1986-87	1987-88	1988-89	1989-90	1990-91	1991-92	1992-93	1993-94	1994-95
All Regions	**29,599**	**27,285**	**26,912**	**30,368**	**35,417**	**38,100**	**41,951**	**44,822**	**45,083**	**44,234**
Public	27,594	25,133	24,832	28,203	32,745	35,294	38,588	41,549	41,039	39,501
Private	2,005	2,152	2,080	2,165	2,672	2,806	3,363	3,273	4,044	4,733
North Atlantic	6,168	5,207	4,856	5,595	6,493	7,175	7,659	8,676	9,058	8,616
Public	5,319	4,397	4,050	4,805	5,399	5,918	6,238	7,314	7,366	6,745
Private	849	810	806	790	1,094	1,257	1,421	1,362	1,692	1,871
Midwest	7,085	6,619	6,839	7,536	9,116	9,651	10,603	11,167	11,308	10,883
Public	6,848	6,295	6,653	7,228	8,781	9,288	10,307	10,962	10,654	10,383
Private	237	324	186	308	335	363	296	205	654	500
South	11,703	10,879	10,693	12,236	14,256	15,708	17,476	18,484	18,663	18,723
Public	11,316	10,444	10,197	11,684	13,543	14,909	16,280	17,225	17,359	17,176
Private	387	435	496	552	713	799	1,196	1,259	1,304	1,547
West	4,643	4,580	4,524	5,001	5,552	5,566	6,213	6,495	6,054	6,012
Public	4,111	3,997	3,932	4,486	5,022	5,179	5,763	6,048	5,660	5,197
Private	532	583	592	515	530	387	450	447	394	815

[1] Excludes American Samoa, Guam, Puerto Rico, and the Virgin Islands.

Table 20
GRADUATIONS FROM LPN/LVN PROGRAMS,
BY NLN REGION AND TYPE OF ADMINISTRATIVE CONTROL: 1985-86 TO 1994-95

NLN REGION BY TYPE OF ADMINISTRATIVE CONTROL [1]	NUMBER OF GRADUATIONS									
	1985-86	1986-87	1987-88	1988-89	1989-90	1990-91	1991-92	1992-93	1993-94	1994-95
All Regions	**29,599**	**27,285**	**26,912**	**30,368**	**35,417**	**38,100**	**41,951**	**44,822**	**45,083**	**44,234**
Technical or vocational school	16,565	14,946	14,608	16,010	18,470	19,755	22,095	24,026	24,229	23,124
Junior or community college	8,784	8,956	9,519	10,797	12,493	14,189	15,235	15,843	15,762	15,611
Secondary school	2,334	1,647	1,476	1,759	2,037	2,044	2,112	2,361	2,598	2,793
Hospital	833	714	782	956	1,273	975	1,118	1,181	1,155	1,114
Government agency	707	747	314	577	830	675	740	718	694	659
Senior college or university	213	93	131	167	167	276	365	417	307	456
Independent agency	163	182	82	102	147	186	286	276	338	477
North Atlantic	6,168	5,207	4,856	5,595	6,493	7,175	7,659	8,676	9,058	8,616
Technical or vocational school	4,112	3,553	3,448	3,754	4,498	4,976	5,414	6,186	6,382	6,195
Junior or community college	615	525	480	734	736	889	954	942	1,018	937
Secondary school	951	724	542	614	637	661	555	785	1,036	654
Hospital	383	304	341	389	509	454	499	522	474	487
Government agency	49	101	45	58	65	73	58	74	53	33
Senior college or university	0	0	0	46	48	122	157	149	77	80
Independent agency	58	0	0	0	0	0	22	18	18	230
Midwest	7,085	6,619	6,839	7,536	9,116	9,651	10,603	11,167	11,308	10,883
Technical or vocational college	3,972	3,529	3,629	3,941	4,802	5,254	5,556	6,088	6,389	5,672
Junior or community college	2,549	2,601	2,789	3,016	3,584	3,917	4,338	4,329	4,333	4,346
Secondary school	455	300	267	428	297	233	558	580	379	674
Hospital	61	57	59	76	85	52	68	66	29	60
Government agency	0	115	48	48	287	133	0	0	47	0
Senior college or university	32	0	33	7	23	20	25	45	65	131
Independent agency	16	17	14	20	38	42	58	59	66	0
South	11,703	10,879	10,693	12,236	14,256	15,708	17,476	18,484	18,663	18,723
Technical or vocational school	6,858	6,470	6,231	6,921	7,662	8,159	9,160	9,382	9,811	9,493
Junior or community college	3,179	3,078	3,458	3,955	4,782	5,814	6,264	6,898	6,636	6,791
Secondary school	524	395	369	358	655	733	615	670	699	942
Hospital	389	353	382	491	632	469	551	593	612	541
Government agency	658	531	201	447	469	457	661	624	585	605
Senior college or university	48	27	24	37	34	36	80	118	96	104
Independent agency	47	25	28	27	22	40	145	199	224	247
West	4,643	4,580	4,524	5,001	5,552	5,566	6,213	6,495	6,054	6,012
Technical or vocational school	1,623	1,394	1,300	1,394	1,508	1,366	1,965	2,370	1,647	1,764
Junior or community college	2,441	2,752	2,792	3,092	3,391	3,569	3,679	3,674	3,775	3,537
Secondary school	404	228	298	359	448	417	384	326	484	523
Hospital	0	0	0	0	47	0	0	0	40	26
Government agency	0	0	20	24	9	12	21	20	9	21
Senior college or university	133	66	74	77	62	98	103	105	69	141
Independent agency	42	140	40	55	87	104	61	0	30	0

[1] Excludes American Samoa, Guam, Puerto Rico, and the Virgin Islands.

157

Table 21
MEAN ANNUAL TUITIONS OF FULL-TIME STUDENTS IN PUBLIC OR PRIVATE LPN/LVN PROGRAMS, BY NLN REGION: 1994-95[1]

| REGION | PRINCIPAL FINANCIAL SUPPORT OF SCHOOL | | |
| | Public | | Private |
	Resident	Non-Resident	
All Regions	**$1,861**	**$3,363**	**$5,834**
North Atlantic	3,397	4,637	5,133
Midwest	2,325	3,644	6,866
South	1,361	2,775	3,558
West	990	3,443	8,919

[1] Excludes American Samoa, Guam, Puerto Rico, and the Virgin Islands.

Table 22
APPLICATIONS PER FALL ADMISSION FOR LPN/LVN PROGRAMS: 1995[1]

REGION[2]	NUMBER OF APPLICATIONS	NUMBER OF FALL ADMISSIONS	APPLICATIONS PER FALL ADMISSION
All Regions	**70,085**	**27,126**	**2.58**
North Altantic	15,875	6,434	2.47
Midwest	16,743	6,927	2.42
South	31,246	11,107	2.81
West	6,221	2,658	2.34

[1] To be included in this tabulation, a nursing program must have answered the question on number of applications and must have admitted a class in the fall of the survey year.
[2] Excludes American Samoa, Guam, Puerto Rico, and the Virgin Islands.

Table 23
PERCENTAGE OF APPLICATIONS FOR ADMISSION ACCEPTED AND NOT ACCEPTED AND PERCENTAGE ON WAITING LISTS FOR ALL LPN/LVN PROGRAMS: 1995

Total Applications[1]	**100.0**
Accepted	41.1
Not Accepted	58.9
Percent of Qualified Applicants Not Accepted and Placed on Waiting Lists	17.0

[1] Excludes American Samoa, Guam, Puerto Rico, and the Virgin Islands.

Section 3-4
Numeric Tables
on Male and Minority Students

Table 1
ESTIMATED NUMBER OF STUDENT ADMISSIONS
TO LPN/LVN PROGRAMS, BY RACE/ETHNICITY, NLN REGION AND STATE: 1994-1995[1]

NLN REGION AND STATE	NUMBER OF PROGRAMS	TOTAL LPN/LVN ADMISSIONS[2]	NUMBER OF ADMISSIONS				
			White	Black	Hispanic	Asian	American Indian
United States	**1,107**	**57,906**	**39,361**	**12,118**	**3,524**	**2,024**	**905**
North Atlantic	176	10,969	7,705	2,389	480	321	81
Midwest	258	13,145	10,200	2,053	380	264	248
South	505	27,400	18,066	6,593	1,752	574	428
West	168	6,392	3,390	1,083	912	865	148
Alabama	22	3,117	2,136	931	14	23	13
Alaska	0	0	0	0	0	0	0
Arizona	13	337	229	24	66	8	10
Arkansas	28	1,016	815	142	27	23	9
California	69	3,580	1,324	795	648	718	101
Colorado	17	442	307	67	47	16	3
Connecticut	12	442	293	95	31	17	7
Delaware	3	165	134	28	0	3	0
District of Columbia	3	256	117	114	15	7	3
Florida	41	3,555	2,196	1,019	219	86	33
Georgia	38	2,278	1,324	779	101	56	20
Hawaii	4	178	89	31	12	46	2
Idaho	5	160	139	9	9	3	1
Illinois	36	2,053	1,363	551	65	70	3
Indiana	22	1,726	1,315	260	85	44	20
Iowa	26	1,042	939	21	35	20	27
Kansas	17	633	525	72	20	11	6
Kentucky	17	1,448	1,162	194	53	30	10
Louisiana	45	2,649	1,716	668	155	82	33
Maine	5	0	0	0	0	0	0
Maryland	11	322	227	86	7	2	1
Massachusetts	20	932	738	153	23	15	3
Michigan	27	758	473	268	9	3	5
Minnesota	24	2,121	1,781	233	20	44	42
Mississippi	15	892	524	285	46	26	8
Missouri	39	1,563	1,277	230	30	17	8
Montana	5	234	201	13	7	3	11
Nebraska	7	365	294	40	19	9	4
Nevada	2	72	63	4	3	2	0
New Hampshire	2	140	140	0	0	0	0
New Jersey	23	1,597	816	518	146	110	10
New Mexico	8	226	138	14	63	9	4
New York	54	4,920	3,440	1,069	230	142	41
North Carolina	31	832	569	198	29	21	16
North Dakota	6	87	52	10	4	2	20
Ohio	41	2,474	1,906	336	85	39	110
Oklahoma	30	1,225	897	121	76	12	120
Oregon	11	42	24	11	4	2	0
Pennsylvania	50	2,433	1,944	412	35	26	17
Rhode Island	1	0	0	0	0	0	0
South Carolina	23	865	572	203	20	14	55
South Dakota	2	63	61	1	0	0	1
Tennessee	26	1,350	978	326	11	8	27
Texas	104	5,378	3,320	1,054	857	116	32
Utah	6	380	279	51	26	14	9
Vermont	3	84	83	0	0	1	0
Virginia	53	1,865	1,185	490	101	53	43
Washington	22	701	557	64	27	44	7
West Virginia	21	608	445	97	36	22	8
Wisconsin	11	260	214	31	8	5	2
Wyoming	6	40	40	0	0	0	0

[1] Excludes American Samoa, Guam, Puerto Rico, and the Virgin Islands.
[2] Due to rounding, the racial/ethnic estimations sometimes add up to slightly more or less than the true total.

Table 2
TRENDS IN THE ESTIMATED NUMBER OF ANNUAL ADMISSIONS
OF MINORITY STUDENTS TO LPN/LVN PROGRAMS: 1990-91 TO 1994-95[1]

YEAR	BLACK		HISPANIC		ASIAN		AMERICAN INDIAN	
	Number	Percent	Number	Percent	Number	Percent	Number	Percent
ALL REGIONS								
1990-91	10,144	18.0	2,416	4.3	1,782	3.2	576	1.0
1991-92	10,524	18.1	2,449	4.2	1,982	3.4	680	1.2
1992-93	12,042	19.8	2,609	4.3	1,852	3.0	562	0.9
1993-94	10,088	16.6	2,837	4.7	1,469	2.4	714	1.2
1994-95	12,118	20.9	3,524	6.1	2,024	3.5	905	1.6
NORTH ATLANTIC								
1990-91	2,243	21.0	258	2.4	136	1.1	25	0.2
1991-92	2,334	20.9	291	2.6	266	2.4	100	0.9
1992-93	2,789	23.4	263	2.2	180	1.5	28	0.2
1993-94	2,164	18.1	380	3.2	176	1.5	46	0.4
1994-95	2,389	21.8	480	4.4	321	2.9	81	0.7
MIDWEST								
1990-91	1,770	12.3	240	1.7	125	0.9	150	1.1
1991-92	1,665	12.3	279	2.1	252	1.9	163	1.2
1992-93	1,784	12.6	305	2.2	172	1.2	160	1.1
1993-94	1,638	11.2	343	2.3	273	1.9	155	1.1
1994-95	2,053	15.6	380	2.9	264	2.0	248	1.9
SOUTH								
1990-91	5,558	22.2	1,135	4.5	207	0.8	266	1.0
1991-92	5,670	21.5	1,103	4.2	495	1.9	294	1.1
1992-93	6,473	23.5	1,272	4.6	444	1.6	257	0.9
1993-94	5,457	19.5	1,404	5.0	531	1.9	402	1.4
1994-95	6,593	24.1	1,752	6.4	574	2.1	428	1.6
WEST								
1990-91	573	8.7	783	11.8	1,314	20.0	135	2.0
1991-92	855	11.9	776	10.8	969	13.5	123	1.7
1992-93	996	13.8	769	10.7	1,056	14.7	117	1.6
1993-94	829	13.6	710	11.6	489	8.0	111	1.8
1994-95	1,083	16.9	912	14.3	865	13.5	148	2.3

[1] Excludes American Samoa, Guam, Puerto Rico, and the Virgin Islands.

Table 3
ESTIMATED NUMBER OF STUDENT ENROLLMENTS
IN LPN/LVN PROGRAMS, BY RACE/ETHNICITY, NLN REGION AND STATE: 1995[1]

NLN REGION AND STATE	NUMBER OF PROGRAMS	TOTAL LPN/LVN ENROLLMENTS[2]	NUMBER OF ENROLLMENTS				
			White	Black	Hispanic	Asian	American Indian
United States	**1,107**	**56,028**	**39,239**	**10,500**	**3,528**	**1,760**	**1,025**
North Atlantic	176	10,877	7,872	2,105	552	256	99
Midwest	258	13,305	10,468	1,849	449	260	284
South	505	25,503	17,048	5,768	1,731	514	449
West	168	6,343	3,851	778	796	730	193
Alabama	22	2,921	1,870	844	123	50	36
Alaska	0	0	0	0	0	0	0
Arizona	13	333	273	18	34	5	3
Arkansas	28	922	766	120	21	10	5
California	69	3,593	1,729	542	569	612	145
Colorado	17	412	304	47	47	6	7
Connecticut	12	457	353	74	20	6	4
Delaware	3	135	94	32	3	4	2
District of Columbia	3	226	48	163	10	2	2
Florida	41	3,214	1,876	931	328	64	14
Georgia	38	2,258	1,451	601	127	50	35
Hawaii	4	228	116	36	17	55	4
Idaho	5	148	131	7	6	2	2
Illinois	36	2,024	1,461	368	102	78	16
Indiana	22	1,820	1,352	303	108	37	24
Iowa	26	1,244	1,128	26	41	22	26
Kansas	17	605	494	55	37	8	12
Kentucky	17	1,180	1,007	115	37	13	10
Louisiana	45	1,955	1,371	453	82	32	19
Maine	5	0	0	0	0	0	0
Maryland	11	377	274	88	8	5	2
Massachusetts	20	966	737	178	32	12	8
Michigan	27	916	632	251	13	9	11
Minnesota	24	2,216	1,824	274	13	47	59
Mississippi	15	891	560	253	47	16	14
Missouri	39	1,435	1,154	227	22	16	18
Montana	5	258	211	24	12	3	7
Nebraska	7	314	265	26	13	4	6
Nevada	2	70	60	1	6	3	0
New Hampshire	2	194	171	15	5	3	1
New Jersey	23	1,858	1,204	429	129	72	25
New Mexico	8	165	92	11	54	5	4
New York	54	4,641	3,267	910	297	131	39
North Carolina	31	824	586	182	27	13	17
North Dakota	6	119	74	13	6	3	23
Ohio	41	2,258	1,791	271	83	25	85
Oklahoma	30	1,167	851	123	23	19	151
Oregon	11	47	38	5	2	1	1
Pennsylvania	50	2,306	1,904	304	56	26	18
Rhode Island	1	0	0	0	0	0	0
South Carolina	23	778	506	209	15	12	34
South Dakota	2	63	61	1	0	0	1
Tennessee	26	1,197	848	315	23	6	6
Texas	104	4,902	3,165	830	766	101	35
Utah	6	369	283	43	25	10	8
Vermont	3	94	94	0	0	0	0
Virginia	53	2,374	1,501	632	72	110	60
Washington	22	681	575	44	24	28	12
West Virginia	21	543	416	72	32	13	11
Wisconsin	11	291	232	34	11	11	3
Wyoming	6	39	39	0	0	0	0

[1] Excludes American Samoa, Guam, Puerto Rico, and the Virgin Islands.
[2] Due to rounding, the racial/ethnic estimations sometimes add up to slightly more or less than the true total.

Table 4
TRENDS IN THE ESTIMATED NUMBER OF ENROLLMENTS
OF MINORITY STUDENTS IN LPN/LVN PROGRAMS: 1990-91 TO 1994-95[1]

YEAR	BLACK		HISPANIC		ASIAN		AMERICAN INDIAN	
	Number	Percent	Number	Percent	Number	Percent	Number	Percent
ALL REGIONS								
1990-91	9,226	16.3	2,252	4.0	1,665	3.0	427	0.8
1991-92	11,206	19.0	2,307	3.9	1,971	3.3	743	1.3
1992-93	11,661	19.1	2,413	4.0	1,639	2.7	731	1.2
1993-94	10,483	17.6	3,373	5.7	1,839	3.1	843	1.4
1994-95	10,500	18.7	3,528	6.3	1,760	3.1	1,025	1.8
NORTH ATLANTIC								
1990-91	2,600	21.4	312	2.6	153	1.3	41	0.3
1991-92	2,831	22.9	277	2.2	318	2.6	92	0.7
1992-93	3,344	25.8	340	2.6	234	1.8	174	1.3
1993-94	2,275	18.3	443	3.6	225	1.8	94	0.8
1994-95	2,105	19.3	552	5.1	256	2.4	99	0.9
MIDWEST								
1990-91	1,399	10.0	243	1.7	167	1.2	115	0.8
1991-92	1,695	12.1	223	1.6	249	1.8	195	1.4
1992-93	1,854	12.5	312	2.1	172	1.2	136	0.9
1993-94	1,822	12.4	499	3.4	357	2.4	294	2.0
1994-95	1,849	13.9	449	3.4	260	2.0	284	2.1
SOUTH								
1990-91	4,722	20.0	1,000	4.8	237	1.0	201	0.8
1991-92	5,883	23.0	993	3.9	418	1.6	303	1.2
1992-93	5,736	22.2	1,101	4.3	389	1.5	259	1.0
1993-94	5,394	20.9	1,681	6.5	680	2.6	329	1.3
1994-95	5,768	22.6	1,731	6.8	514	2.0	449	1.8
WEST								
1990-91	505	7.5	697	10.4	1,108	16.5	70	1.0
1991-92	797	11.2	814	11.4	986	13.8	153	2.1
1992-93	727	9.9	660	9.0	844	11.5	162	2.2
1993-94	992	15.0	750	11.4	577	8.7	126	1.9
1994-95	778	12.3	796	12.5	730	11.5	193	3.0

[1] Excludes American Samoa, Guam, Puerto Rico, and the Virgin Islands.

NLN REGION AND STATE	NUMBER OF PROGRAMS	TOTAL LPN/LVN GRADUATIONS[2]	NUMBER OF GRADUATIONS				
			White	Black	Hispanic	Asian	American Indian
United States	**1,107**	**44,234**	**32,650**	**6,954**	**2,431**	**1,531**	**651**
North Atlantic	176	8,616	6,489	1,457	340	259	76
Midwest	258	10,883	8,961	1,185	305	257	172
South	505	18,723	13,345	3,551	1,086	431	295
West	168	6,012	3,855	761	700	584	108
Alabama	22	1,718	1,127	503	42	35	11
Alaska	0	0	0	0	0	0	0
Arizona	13	472	386	17	54	8	5
Arkansas	28	665	552	77	17	13	5
California	69	2,735	1,244	547	446	438	61
Colorado	17	579	448	46	59	17	4
Connecticut	12	395	306	57	17	13	5
Delaware	3	79	62	14	0	3	0
District of Columbia	3	236	115	87	16	12	4
Florida	41	2,503	1,611	666	140	60	26
Georgia	38	1,286	866	301	58	41	15
Hawaii	4	189	102	30	13	41	4
Idaho	5	142	134	2	4	2	2
Illinois	36	1,563	1,269	168	51	68	7
Indiana	22	1,380	1,044	200	69	47	21
Iowa	26	977	930	10	16	8	9
Kansas	17	598	504	55	19	10	7
Kentucky	17	1,057	851	124	40	30	12
Louisiana	45	1,271	913	245	53	41	17
Maine	5	34	29	3	1	1	0
Maryland	11	331	238	76	9	7	3
Massachusetts	20	762	626	98	21	13	4
Michigan	27	1,027	837	145	24	15	7
Minnesota	24	1,296	1,043	195	12	23	22
Mississippi	15	699	463	167	33	25	9
Missouri	39	1,273	1,099	123	23	18	9
Montana	5	134	104	13	7	5	5
Nebraska	7	315	253	29	14	13	7
Nevada	2	99	75	11	7	5	1
New Hampshire	2	108	90	9	5	3	1
New Jersey	23	1,268	739	369	60	91	9
New Mexico	8	236	155	9	63	5	3
New York	54	3,254	2,402	535	179	99	44
North Carolina	31	655	504	101	24	16	9
North Dakota	6	143	116	11	6	3	8
Ohio	41	1,996	1,608	218	58	43	71
Oklahoma	30	887	688	83	11	6	99
Oregon	11	201	181	5	5	4	7
Pennsylvania	50	2,333	1,998	272	35	19	7
Rhode Island	1	63	39	13	6	4	2
South Carolina	23	546	381	114	8	9	33
South Dakota	2	58	56	1	0	0	1
Tennessee	26	949	724	197	7	16	4
Texas	104	4,503	3,253	601	564	61	15
Utah	6	401	318	37	21	16	9
Vermont	3	84	83	0	0	1	0
Virginia	53	1,132	780	229	52	47	25
Washington	22	726	622	39	17	41	5
West Virginia	21	521	394	67	28	24	12
Wisconsin	11	257	202	30	13	9	3
Wyoming	6	98	86	5	4	2	2

[1] Excludes American Samoa, Guam, Puerto Rico, and the Virgin Islands.
[2] Due to rounding, the racial/ethnic estimations sometimes add up to slightly more or less than the true total.

Table 6
TRENDS IN THE ESTIMATED NUMBER OF GRADUATIONS
OF MINORITY STUDENTS FROM LPN/LVN PROGRAMS: 1990-91 TO 1994-95[1]

YEAR	BLACK		HISPANIC		ASIAN		AMERICAN INDIAN	
	Number	Percent	Number	Percent	Number	Percent	Number	Percent
ALL REGIONS								
1990-91	5,421	14.2	1,720	4.5	956	2.5	260	0.7
1991-92	6,575	15.7	1,628	3.9	1,329	3.2	415	1.0
1992-93	7,785	17.4	2,298	5.1	1,115	2.5	363	0.8
1993-94	6,463	14.3	1,942	4.3	1,594	3.5	453	1.0
1994-95	6,954	15.7	2,431	5.5	1,531	3.5	651	1.5
NORTH ATLANTIC								
1990-91	1,324	18.5	156	2.2	80	1.1	8	0.1
1991-92	1,368	17.9	194	2.5	185	2.4	56	0.7
1992-93	1,839	21.2	295	3.4	113	1.3	24	0.3
1993-94	1,503	16.6	258	2.8	184	2.0	40	0.4
1994-95	1,457	16.9	340	3.9	259	3.0	76	0.9
MIDWEST								
1990-91	845	8.6	175	1.8	111	1.6	49	0.5
1991-92	1,161	10.9	188	1.8	170	1.6	79	0.7
1992-93	1,138	10.2	288	2.6	131	1.2	49	0.4
1993-94	1,037	9.2	216	1.9	252	2.2	85	0.7
1994-95	1,185	10.9	305	2.8	257	2.4	172	1.6
SOUTH								
1990-91	2,892	18.4	825	5.3	156	5.6	134	0.9
1991-92	3,314	19.0	659	3.8	252	1.4	149	0.8
1992-93	4,248	23.0	901	4.9	214	1.2	166	0.9
1993-94	3,176	17.0	954	5.1	546	2.9	258	1.4
1994-95	3,551	19.0	1,086	5.8	431	2.3	295	1.6
WEST								
1990-91	360	6.7	564	10.1	609	10.9	69	1.2
1991-92	732	11.8	587	9.4	722	11.6	131	2.1
1992-93	560	8.6	814	12.5	657	10.1	124	1.9
1993-94	747	12.3	514	8.5	612	10.1	70	1.2
1994-95	761	12.7	700	11.7	584	9.7	108	1.8

[1] Excludes American Samoa, Guam, Puerto Rico, and the Virgin Islands.

Table 7
ADMISSIONS OF MEN TO LPN/LVN PROGRAMS,
BY NLN REGION: 1994-1995[1]

NLN REGION	NUMBER OF PROGRAMS REPORTING	TOTAL ADMISSIONS	MEN	
			Number	Percent
All Regions	**652**	**38,377**	**4,553**	**11.9**
North Atlantic	123	7,376	767	10.4
Midwest	165	9,616	931	9.7
South	292	17,846	2,296	12.9
West	72	3,539	559	15.8

[1] Excludes American Samoa, Guam, Puerto Rico, and the Virgin Islands.

Table 8
TRENDS IN ADMISSIONS OF MEN
TO LPN/LVN PROGRAMS: 1985-1995[1,2]

YEAR	NUMBER OF PROGRAMS REPORTING	MEN	
		Number	Percent
ALL REGIONS			
1985	851	2,167	6.1
1987	738	1,862	6.1
1988	780	2,602	7.8
1989	1,026	2,860	6.0
1991	571	3,386	9.7
1992	674	4,038	9.9
1993	633	4,981	12.5
1994	671	5,499	13.0
1995	652	4,553	11.9
NORTH ATLANTIC			
1985	158	513	6.1
1987	135	266	4.5
1988	146	363	5.5
1989	179	489	5.4
1991	112	595	8.7
1992	135	874	9.8
1993	116	937	11.1
1994	128	1,041	12.3
1995	123	767	10.4
MIDWEST			
1985	199	517	6.0
1987	181	505	6.2
1988	181	443	5.4
1989	222	599	5.3
1991	151	824	8.1
1992	170	1,013	9.6
1993	162	1,171	11.4
1994	175	1,187	10.3
1995	165	931	9.7
SOUTH			
1985	368	757	5.3
1987	314	726	6.0
1988	348	1,365	9.5
1989	464	1,383	6.6
1991	252	1,661	10.9
1992	294	1,569	9.2
1993	291	2,167	12.8
1994	295	2,545	13.8
1995	292	2,296	12.9
WEST			
1985	126	380	9.2
1987	108	365	8.9
1988	105	431	10.5
1989	161	389	6.3
1991	56	306	11.2
1992	75	582	14.7
1993	64	706	17.2
1994	73	726	18.2
1995	72	559	15.8

[1] Excludes American Samoa, Guam, Puerto Rico, and the Virgin Islands.
[2] No data is available for 1986 and 1990.

Table 9
ENROLLMENTS OF MEN IN LPN/LVN PROGRAMS, BY NLN REGION: 1995[1]

NLN REGION	NUMBER OF PROGRAMS REPORTING	TOTAL ENROLLMENTS	MEN	
			Number	Percent
All Regions	**629**	**34,020**	**3,934**	**11.6**
North Atlantic	118	6,241	653	10.5
Midwest	155	8,682	790	9.1
South	286	15,757	1,993	12.6
West	70	3,340	498	14.9

[1] Excludes American Samoa, Guam, Puerto Rico, and the Virgin Islands.

Table 10
TRENDS IN ENROLLMENTS OF MEN IN LPN/LVN PROGRAMS: 1985-1995[1,2]

YEAR	NUMBER OF PROGRAMS REPORTING	MEN	
		Number	Percent
ALL REGIONS			
1985	851	1,664	5.6
1988	779	2,568	7.8
1989	1,026	2,654	5.7
1991	581	3,416	10.0
1992	692	4,198	9.9
1993	617	4,534	11.9
1994	668	5,022	12.6
1995	629	3,934	11.6
NORTH ATLANTIC			
1985	158	423	5.7
1988	146	403	5.9
1989	179	428	4.5
1991	115	651	8.8
1992	134	989	10.2
1993	118	986	10.7
1994	128	943	10.4
1995	118	653	10.5
MIDWEST			
1985	199	375	5.3
1988	180	410	4.9
1989	222	568	5.0
1991	155	780	8.0
1992	168	962	9.0
1993	160	948	9.5
1994	171	1,086	10.3
1995	155	790	9.1
SOUTH			
1985	368	583	4.9
1988	348	1,389	10.1
1989	464	1,312	6.8
1991	248	1,539	11.2
1992	312	1,698	9.5
1993	274	1,935	13.0
1994	299	2,355	14.2
1995	286	1,993	12.6
WEST			
1985	126	283	8.2
1988	105	366	9.4
1989	161	346	5.3
1991	63	446	13.2
1992	78	549	14.3
1993	65	665	17.3
1994	70	638	17.1
1995	70	498	14.9

[1] Excludes American Samoa, Guam, Puerto Rico, and the Virgin Islands.
[2] No data is available for 1986, 1987 and 1990.

Table 11
GRADUATIONS OF MEN FROM LPN/LVN PROGRAMS,
BY NLN REGION: 1994-1995[1]

NLN REGION	NUMBER OF PROGRAMS REPORTING	TOTAL GRADUATIONS	MEN	
			Number	Percent
All Regions	**645**	**28,110**	**3,536**	**12.6**
North Atlantic	119	5,515	616	11.2
Midwest	164	7,178	702	9.8
South	274	11,948	1,657	13.9
West	88	3,469	561	16.2

[1] Excludes American Samoa, Guam, Puerto Rico, and the Virgin Islands.

Table 12
TRENDS IN GRADUATIONS OF MEN
FROM LPN/LVN PROGRAMS: 1985-1995[1,2]

YEAR	NUMBER OF PROGRAMS REPORTING	MEN	
		Number	Percent
ALL REGIONS			
1985	851	1,372	4.9
1988	782	1,184	5.8
1989	1,041	1,608	5.3
1991	551	2,103	9.4
1992	639	2,707	9.4
1993	599	3,060	11.1
1994	656	3,910	12.8
1995	645	3,536	12.6
NORTH ATLANTIC			
1985	158	250	4.0
1988	147	208	5.3
1989	179	219	3.9
1991	110	337	7.4
1992	115	503	9.0
1993	114	603	10.1
1994	125	745	11.1
1995	119	616	11.2
MIDWEST			
1985	199	312	4.1
1988	181	212	4.0
1989	234	349	4.6
1991	147	493	7.8
1992	164	620	7.8
1993	159	635	8.3
1994	168	805	9.6
1995	164	702	9.8
SOUTH			
1985	368	503	4.7
1988	349	516	6.3
1989	466	781	6.4
1991	231	1,007	10.9
1992	264	1,047	9.2
1993	243	1,318	12.8
1994	272	1,776	15.0
1995	274	1,657	13.9
WEST			
1985	126	307	7.6
1988	105	248	8.6
1989	162	259	5.2
1991	63	266	11.7
1992	96	537	13.7
1993	83	504	14.0
1994	91	584	16.0
1995	88	561	16.2

[1] Excludes American Samoa, Guam, Puerto Rico, and the Virgin Islands.
[2] No data is available for 1986, 1987 and 1990.